The Applicant's Manual

OF PHYSICIAN ASSISTANT PROGRAMS

Mark Volpe, PA-C

Brittany Hogan

The Applicant's Manual of Physician Assistant Programs

1st Edition

ISBN-13: 978-1519198112

ISBN-10: 1519198116

Notice: PA program admissions is an ever-changing process. Every effort has been made to ensure that the information in this book is up to date and accurate. However, given the possibility of human error and changes in admissions processes, neither the authors nor the publisher no any other party who has been involved in the preparation or publication of this work warrants that the information contained herein is in every respect accurate or complete, and they disclaim all responsibility for any errors or omissions or for the results obtained from use of the information contained in this work. Readers are encouraged to confirm the information contained herein with other sources.

About the Author:

Mark Volpe, MPH, MMSc, PA-C is a physician assistant practicing in outpatient internal medicine and urgent care in Connecticut. He graduated from the Yale University PA Program in 2015, where he played a role in several aspects of the admissions process throughout three admissions cycles. He completed his MPH from Southern Connecticut State University and his BS from the University of Connecticut. He has particular interest in PA program admissions, education, and physician assistant research. During his time at Yale he was published in several peer-reviewed journals, completed a medical education elective, and also was awarded both the Paul Ambrose Fellowship through the Association for Prevention Teaching and Research as well as the Future Educator Fellowship through the Physician Assistant Education Association.

Contributor:

Brittany Hogan, PA-S is a second year PA student at Yale University. Brittany earned her BS from Fordham University in 2010. She then spent a few years working in New York City as an EEG technician and then in Boston as a weight loss coach. After meeting and shadowing PAs during that time, Brittany discovered that the profession was a perfect fit for her. In her limited free time Brittany enjoys soccer, running, writing, painting, and cooking. Brittany plans to move to the Boston area after graduating and hopes to work in Dermatology or Plastic Surgery.

TABLE OF CONTENTS

INTRODUCTION

Purpose

Welcome to *The Applicant's Manual of Physician Assistant Programs*. This guide was formulated for prospective students applying to physician assistant (PA) programs and provides specific, pertinent, detailed information about each accredited PA program in the United States as of January 2016. Applicants should use this guide as a primary resource to investigate each program and evaluate their credentials relative to those typically desired by each program. This guide is the first of its kind to incorporate all relevant information about each PA program into a single reference, saving the applicant the substantial amount of time it typically takes to explore multiple programs. This guide also provides the applicant with a quick and easy resource that can be referenced throughout the application process.

In the coming pages, we will provide an overview of the PA profession, describe the types of information included in this manual, define key terms used throughout the manual, and provide tips for applicants as they navigate the application process. Additionally, we have included reference links where you can find more information about the topics explored throughout the manual. We hope that you find this to be a useful tool throughout the application process.

Overview of the PA Profession

According to the American Academy of Physician Assistants (AAPA), a PA is a nationally certified and state-licensed medical professional. PAs practice medicine on healthcare teams with physicians and other providers. They practice in all medical specialties and prescribe medication in all 50 states, the District of Columbia, the majority of the U.S. territories and the uniformed services. PAs work in collaboration with physicians and other providers as part of the healthcare team to provide high-quality care to patients.

Though the duties of a PA can vary based on their practice setting, experience, and chosen specialty, PAs are trained to perform many of the same tasks as their physician counterparts including (1) taking a medical history; (2) performing a physical exam; (3) ordering and interpreting laboratory and imaging tests; (4) diagnosing and treating acute and chronic disease; (5) counseling patients; (6) assisting in simple and complex surgery; (7) writing prescriptions; and (8) rounding on patients in hospitals, nursing homes, and other settings. Additionally, some duties of PAs vary based upon state-specific practice laws. In each state, PAs designate a physician whom they collaborate with in the workplace and can utilize as a resource as needed to ensure appropriate patient care.

PAs are educated in PA programs sponsored by colleges and universities throughout the United States and accredited by the Accreditation Review Commission on Education for the Physician Assistant (ARC-PA). The ARC-PA sets standards (referred to as "the Standards") that PA programs must meet to remain accredited and thoroughly evaluates each program to ensure a quality educational experience for all PA students. Each PA program is approximately 24-36 months in duration and most award Master's degrees. In the didactic (classroom) phase, programs provide students with education in basic science, behavioral science, clinical medicine, pathophysiology, pharmacology, anatomy, physiology, history taking, physical diagnosis and much more. In the clinical phase, students complete over 2,000 hours of rotations in a variety of settings and specialties which include primary care, internal medicine, obstetrics and gynecology, pediatrics, surgery, emergency medicine, and psychiatry. Most PA programs also have elective rotations that students can participate in to further their knowledge in a particular area of medicine. Examples of elective rotations include dermatology, orthopedics, endocrinology, cardiology, and many others. Thus, PAs upon graduation are well-trained generalists, with foundational knowledge in several areas of medicine that they can then use to practice general internal medicine or enter into any specialty of their choosing.

After completing a PA Program, students then take the Physician Assistant National Certification Exam (PANCE), which is created by the National Commission on the Certification of Physician Assistants (NCCPA). Once the PANCE is successfully completed, the credential of physician assistant – certified (PA-C) is utilized by PAs to denote their certification by the NCCPA. Before practicing, PAs then must complete licensing requirements in the state with which they wish to practice. Subsequently, PAs then complete continuing medical education credits throughout their career as well as recertification exams to maintain their proficiency and competency in general medicine. This allows PAs to maintain their certified status and also ensures that the PA maintains the requisite general medical knowledge to be able to transition into different specialties throughout their career if desired.

Currently, the PA profession is in a stage of unprecedented growth. There are over 190 currently accredited PA programs in the United States, up from 136 accredited programs just 10 years ago. By 2020 it is projected that there will be over 250 PA programs. The job growth in the United States from 2014-2024 for PAs is predicted at over 30%, which is much faster than the national average. Additionally, the median annual compensation for a PA in the United States in 2014 was $95,820. The PA profession is also expanding internationally to countries such as England, Canada, and Australia among others, where new educational programs under different accrediting bodies and standards are beginning to train PAs to practice in those countries.

Links for Further Information

- American Academy of Physician Assistants: www.aapa.org
- Accreditation Review Commission on Education for the Physician Assistant: www. arc-pa.org
- International Academy of Physician Associate Educators: www.iapae.com
- National Commission on the Certification of Physician Assistants: www.nccpa.net
- United States Department of Labor: www.bls.gov/ooh/healthcare/physician-assistants.htm

IMPORTANT ADMISSIONS INFORMATION

Overview

This section will provide a review of the information provided about each accredited physician assistant program in subsequent pages. The goal of this section is to help you understand the information given about each school, provide you with general information about PA admissions, and also provide you with tips on navigating the admissions process to put yourself in the best position to succeed. We also provide links and resources for further information.

Contact Information

For each school, we provide detailed contact information. This includes the mailing address, primary phone contact, and primary email contact. This information should be used as your primary means of communicating with programs when you have general program questions, questions about the application process or your specific application, and for submitting any additional information that programs may require. Such information may include official transcripts, updated course grades and GPAs if courses were in progress at the time of application, or updates to other sections of your application such as healthcare experience, awards, research, certifications, or others.

Program Highlights

In this section, we provide information about the accreditation status, degree offered, start date, program length, class capacity, and tuition for each PA program.

Accreditation

PA programs are accredited by the ARC-PA and given one of several different accreditation statuses listed below:

(1) **Accreditation – Provisional** is an accreditation status granted when the plans and resource allocation, if fully implemented as planned, of a proposed program that has not yet enrolled students appear to demonstrate the program's ability to meet the ARC-PA *Standards* or when a program holding accreditation-provisional status appears to demonstrate continued progress in complying with the *Standards* as it prepares for the graduation of the first class (cohort) of students. Accreditation - Provisional does not ensure any subsequent accreditation status. Accreditation - Provisional is limited to no more than five

years from matriculation of the first class. PA students who attend programs that are provisionally accredited on admission are able to sit for the PANCE upon graduation.

(2) **Accreditation – Continued** is granted (1) when a currently accredited program is in compliance with the Standards, (2) in the case of a program holding Accreditation-Probation when the program has demonstrated that it is once again in compliance with the Standards, or (3) when a program holding Accreditation-Provisional demonstrates compliance with the *Standards* after completion of the provisional review process. Accreditation-continued status remains in effect until the program closes or withdraws from the accreditation process or until accreditation is withdrawn for failure to comply with the Standards.

(3) **Accreditation – Probation** is a temporary status of accreditation, limited to two years, granted when a program holding an accreditation status of accreditation-provisional or accreditation-continued does not meet the *Standards* and when the capability of the program to provide an acceptable educational experience for its students is threatened. Once placed on probation, a program that fails to comply with accreditation requirements in a timely manner, as specified by the ARC-PA, may be scheduled for a focused site visit and/or risk having its accreditation withdrawn. Programs that are placed on probation are required to teach out current students that are in the program, even if accreditation is lost, or find other programs willing to accept their students so that they can graduate and sit for the PANCE.

(4) **Accreditation – Administrative** Probation is a temporary status granted when a program has not complied with an administrative requirement, such as failure to pay fees or submit required reports. Once placed on Administrative Probation, a program that fails to comply with administrative requirements in a timely manner, as specified by the ARC-PA, may be scheduled for a focused site visit and/or risk having its accreditation withdrawn.

(5) **Accreditation Withheld** is a status granted when an entry-level program, seeking accreditation-provisional status, is not in compliance with the Standards. The program receiving this accreditation status may voluntarily withdraw from the accreditation process within the 30-day appeal timeframe.

(6) **Accreditation Withdrawn** is a status granted when an established program is determined no longer to be in compliance with the *Standards* and is no longer capable of providing an acceptable educational experience for its students, or when the program has failed to comply with ARC-PA accreditation requirements, actions or procedures. The program may voluntarily withdraw from the accreditation process within the 30-day appeal timeframe.

Degree Offered

The degree status is an important consideration for students applying to PA programs. This section describes the degree that students will receive upon graduation from a given program. As of 2020, all PA programs will be required to offer a Master's degree as the degree conferred upon graduation. However, currently there are 189 programs that offer a Master's degrees, six that offer a Bachelor's degree, two that offer an Associate's degree, and three that offer a Certificate. A student graduating from any accredited PA program, regardless of degree offered, is eligible to take the PANCE in order to become a certified physician assistant upon passing the exam. However, it is becoming increasingly common for PA employment job listings to state that a Master's degree is preferred or required. For prospective PA students who already have a Master's degree or higher, the degree offered by the PA program may be of no consequence. However, for those who do not have a graduate degree, there is the potential for the awarded degree to influence future employment opportunities.

Program Start Date

Additionally, the **start date** of the program is important to consider when selecting PA programs. The majority of programs start in August, January, or May each year. Even still, there are others that start in other months. This becomes important for several reasons. If you are a student who is applying during senior year of undergraduate studies in 2016 for admission to PA Programs, you may be eligible for programs that start in May 2016, August 2016, and January 2017. Some students prefer a break after undergraduate studies, and so may not wish to apply to programs that start in May 2016, immediately after their undergraduate education would end. Others may not want to wait seven months to start a program in January 2017, and so instead should apply to programs with earlier start dates. Furthermore, regardless of whether you are a current undergraduate or have been out of school for several years, you may be accepted to programs with varying start dates and will need to consider the timing of the program start date, its length, your current employment position and finances, as well as potential future lost PA wages if you opt for a program that has a longer duration or a later start date.

Program Length

The **program length** is also an essential consideration in evaluating PA programs. Most PA programs are 24-36 months in duration. There are pros and cons for both shorter and longer programs. In general, longer programs tend to have more built-in breaks and may offer a slightly lighter per-semester course load given the extra time available to complete coursework compared to shorter, more condensed programs. Though longer programs may offer a seemingly better school-life balance, you may also find them attached to a steep price tag. Many programs justify a longer period of training with higher tuition. Attending a longer program will also put you into the workforce later than you might otherwise enter if you attended a shorter program. This may be significant for some, especially if you consider the months to a year of lost wages that you would have begun earning sooner had you attended a shorter program. Choosing program length is largely a personalized decision based on the above-mentioned and other individual factors.

Class Capacity

Another important component of choosing a PA program is its **class capacity**. The class capacity is the maximum amount of students that a PA program is accredited to enroll per class. Most programs tend to fill their class capacity, but not all do. As an example, Yale is accredited to have a class size of up to 45 students per year, however routinely selects 36-40 students. Programs have class capacities that range from 20-100+ students. Some students are more comfortable in a smaller, more intimate program, while other students may prefer larger, more robust learning environments. Regardless of your preference, it is important to be aware of the size of the program. If you are unsure whether you prefer a larger or smaller program, you should apply to both smaller and larger programs and then evaluate each when you visit campus for interviews, information sessions, or other prospective student events.

Tuition

Lastly, in the program highlights we provide you with the **tuition** of each program. Tuition can vary based on several factors, such as whether the institution is public or private, the institution location, and program resources, among others. We provide you solely with the tuition in this manual. We do not include the other PA school expenses such as books, university fees, and living expenses for several reasons. Students can mitigate projected expenses in a variety of ways, such as living at home or on a budget, using savings, getting financial help from family/friends, etc. Thus, projected expenses provided by each school may not be an accurate depiction of what the overall cost will actually be. This will significantly impact the overall cost of PA school. Additionally, many students choose not to buy some or all of the books recommended by each of the programs. Some programs offer all local rotations, while others require significant travel to rotations at an added expense. Thus, the only factor that we could fairly compare that all students would have to pay equally was the tuition. Applicants should utilize the tuition information provided to be able to compare tuitions at different programs, but should also research projected cost of living, university fees, books, scholarships and other financial aid opportunities available at different institutions.

Links for Further Information

- Accreditation Review Commission on Education for the Physician Assistant: www.arc-pa.org
- Physician Assistant Education Association Program Directory: www.directory.paeaonline.org

Student Stats

In this section we provide the most recent statistics for students accepted into each PA program. Some programs report only some or none of these statistics, and so they are not always available for each program. However, for those programs that do report statistics, applicants can compare their statistics to those of the average accepted student to get a gestalt of how likely or unlikely they are to receive an interview and ultimately be accepted to a given program.

For each program we report the **percentage of male and female students** per class as well as the **percentage of minority students** in each class. We also report the average **overall GPA** and **science GPA** for accepted students. These numbers are largely determined by the Central Application Service for Physician Assistants (CASPA), the common application that most PA applicants apply to PA programs through, and may vary slightly from the GPAs that are reported on your undergraduate or graduate transcripts for several reasons. Firstly, CASPA may use a different formula from the undergraduate or graduate institution that you attended to determine GPA. Secondly, CASPA does not accept grade replacement, which some undergraduate and graduate institutions do. This means that if you repeated a course that you performed poorly in and attained a better grade, both the initial grade and the grade on the second attempt will be included in your GPA calculations.

In addition, the average **Graduate Record Examination (GRE)** scores for the quantitative, verbal, and writing sections are reported. Importantly, not all schools require this examination as a part of their admissions requirement. However, it is a good idea to consider taking this exam as it will open up many more opportunities for programs that you can apply to. Additionally, many programs have cutoff values for the GRE, meaning that students who fail to attain a given score automatically will not be interviewed. Typically this score is around 300 total, or the 50th percentile overall. The degree to which programs emphasize GRE scores in their admissions decisions varies, but it is in your best interest to prepare well so that you can maximize this score, particularly if your application is weak in other areas. Finally, we also provide the **student to faculty ratio** for each program, which may be an indicator of how much individualized attention is provided to each student.

Links for Further Information

- Central Application Service for Physician Assistants: https://portal.caspaonline.org/caspaHelpPages/about-caspaoverview/index.html
- Graduate Record Examination: www.gre.org

Application Basics

Types of Admissions

There are several basic components of the application process that each applicant should know about for the schools they are interested in applying to. Schools generally offer one of two types of admissions: rolling or non-rolling. **Rolling admissions** refers to schools that review each application as it is received and in the order that it is received to determine which applicants will receive an invitation to interview. This means that students who apply early in the application cycle are at an advantage compared to those who apply closer to the deadline because their applications will be evaluated sooner in the review process. Students who apply close to the deadline may not receive an interview simply because all of the spots have already been taken. Alternatively, they could be offered an interview to get onto the program's waiting list, rather than to be a part of the next incoming class of students. **Non-rolling admissions** refers to schools that review all of the applications equally and without regard to when they were submitted (as long as they were received prior to the deadline). For these programs, there is no advantage for a student who applies early compared to a student that applies close to the deadline as all applications are reviewed prior to decisions being made about interview spots.

The Common Application

Secondly, applicants need to consider whether or not a program participates in CASPA, the centralized application service. By using **CASPA**, you are able to complete one application online and send one set of documents (transcripts, letters of recommendation) to them. CASPA will verify your coursework for accuracy, calculate your GPA, and submit your application and attached documents to your designated PA programs. You will also be able to enter your personal statement, describing why you want to be a PA, into CASPA. Approximately 90% of programs participate in CASPA. If a program does not participate in CASPA, students need to submit a separate application (and fee) for that program, which may have different content than the CASPA application. It is highly recommended that students review all of the "Before Applying" materials on the CASPA website prior to beginning their application. It is also important to note that once your application is submitted to CASPA, it needs to be verified before it is sent off to the programs as a completed application. This process can take 2-4 weeks and should be taken into consideration to ensure that applicants meet the appropriate deadlines for each school. Further detailed discussion about CASPA is beyond the scope of this text however the CASPA website has detailed information for all applicants and offers customer service for individual questions.

Secondary Applications

Moreover, applicants also need to investigate whether or not a program requires a **secondary application** (and fee). These are applications that are created by some PA programs that students must complete in addition to CASPA. They generally ask questions that are specific to a particular program's mission, interests, and goals. They also may include sections where applicants list the courses they are using to fulfill prerequisites, attach a curriculum vitae, or document other program-specific requirements. Since secondary applications often include essay-style questions, these applications can be time consuming. It is important to plan ahead to complete this application prior to the application deadline for each program.

Application Deadlines

Finally, applicants should be aware of the **application deadline**. We provide the application deadline listed on the program website. However, it is important to realize that there are several different types of application deadlines, which are color coded on the CASPA application. Some programs have e-submission deadlines. This means that if you submit your application to CASPA by the program deadline, you have met the deadline for your application, even though CASPA typically takes another 2-4 weeks to process and verify your application. Other programs have complete date deadlines. This means that in order for applicants to meet the deadline, they must have all transcripts, letters of recommendation and other supporting documents submitted to and received by CASPA prior to the deadline. However, the application does not need to be verified (GPA calculated) by CASPA by the deadline for programs with complete date deadlines. Finally, there are programs with verified deadlines, meaning that all supporting documentation and GPA calculations must be completed by CASPA prior to the program deadline.

Links for Further Information

- Central Application Service for Physician Assistants: https://portal.caspaonline.org/caspaHelpPages/about-caspaoverview/index.html

Application Requirements

Grade Point Average

As expected, every PA program has specific requirements that must be met for admission. Most programs require a 3.0 overall GPA and/or 3.0 science GPA. In order to be a competitive applicant, you should look to exceed both values for your overall and science GPA. Chances are that if your GPA values are less than these minimums, most PA programs will not consider your application for admission to be viable. As previously stated, courses that were taken multiple times will have both the initial and subsequent grades included in these GPA calculations. Furthermore, PA programs also do consider trends in GPAs. A student who steadily improved their GPA from a 2.5 freshman year to a 4.0 senior year is generally viewed more favorably than those who started out with a 4.0 freshman year and then declined to a 2.5 senior year, even though they may have the same overall and science GPA.

Prerequisite Coursework

Moreover, PA programs have specific **prerequisite courserequirements**. We have listed these for each program, as well as any other specific information about those prerequisites. Common courses that many programs require include college-level biology, chemistry, organic chemistry, biochemistry, microbiology, genetics, human anatomy, human physiology, psychology, and statistics. Of course, these vary by program. One common example is that most programs require two semesters of human anatomy and physiology. Most programs will allow you to complete this as either one course in human anatomy and a second course in human physiology, or a two semester sequence of human anatomy and physiology if the courses were not offered as separate entities at your previous school.

Some programs also impose time limits on these courses, meaning that students must have taken the courses in the last 5 years or 10 years, as an example, in order for them to meet the requirement for that given school. If the course was taken in the distant past, students may need to repeat that course again for these programs. Additionally, some programs will allow students to apply while prerequisite courses are still in progress, while others require that all courses be completed prior to application. In general, the more prerequisites completed prior to application the better because programs can more accurately and completely assess your application if more prerequisite grades are available. Finally, programs differ in terms of what types of college credits they will accept. Many programs, for example, accept community college credits, while others do not. Some programs may accept online coursework, Advanced Placement (AP) courses from high school, or course waivers while others do not. Though we have attempted to include this information throughout the text for each school, it is in the applicant's best interest to review this information on the program website for the schools they are interested in, especially if your prerequisites were completed in a non-traditional manner.

Prerequisite Healthcare Experience

In addition to coursework prerequisites, programs have varying levels of required prerequisite **healthcare experience**. Generally, there are two categories of healthcare experience that programs evaluate. The first is direct patient care experience. This refers to experience where applicants were directly responsible for patient care. Often times, these experiences require a certification. Some examples include medical assistant, emergency medical technician, certified nursing assistant, physical therapy aide, physical therapist, registered nurse, emergency department technician, athletic trainer, paramedic, military medic, and many more. PA Programs require anywhere from 0-4000+ hours of direct patient contact experience, and in general the more experience you have, the better your chances are as an applicant, even to programs that require little to no experience. Typically, paid experience is preferred over volunteer experience, as it usually indicates a higher level of responsibility. That being said, many programs do highly value volunteer experiences, both related to and not related to healthcare. Such positions should be sought out, coveted, and confidently reported in the application. By acquiring more experience, you make yourself a competitive applicant for more programs, especially those that have a high number of required healthcare hours.

The second type of healthcare experience is healthcare related experience. These are positions where applicants were performing a role related to healthcare but that did not involve direct patient contact. Examples include medical secretary, office manager, pharmaceutical sales representative, hospital volunteer, pharmacy technician, medical scribe, and others. It is important to note that the definition of what counts as direct patient contact versus healthcare related experience can sometimes vary by program. If you are unsure which category your experience counts for, you should contact the program directly to inquire. For positions where there was a combination of direct patient care responsibility and non-patient care responsibilities, hours worked can be divided into each of those categories on CASPA. As an example, if you worked 2,000 hours as a medical assistant, with 50% of your time devoted to patient care and 50% of your time devoted to clerical work, you would count 1,000 of those hours as direct patient care hours and 1,000 of those hours as healthcare related experience on CASPA. Additionally, many PA programs value and encourage shadowing a PA to learn the role and responsibilities of the profession and to ensure that you are pursuing a career that fits well with your goals and expectations.

Standardized Testing

Also, some programs have **required standardized testing**, while others do not. The most common standardized test requirement for PA programs is the GRE. As previously stated, it is a good idea to consider taking this exam as it will open up many more opportunities for programs that you can apply to as an applicant. Additionally, many programs have cutoff values for the GRE, meaning that if students fail to attain a given score they automatically will not be interviewed. Typically this score is around 300 total, or the 50th percentile overall. Some programs will accept the Medical College Admissions Test (MCAT) in lieu of the GRE, while other programs require the GRE but may waive the requirement if the applicant has a previously attained graduate degree. We have included this information on each school specific page.

Letters of Recommendation

Lastly, **letters of recommendation** are a crucial component of the PA admissions application. Most schools will require 2-3 letters, and some schools have specific requirements as to whom the letters must be written by. Generally, family members, friends, and personal medical providers are not appropriate for writing letters for PA school. Commonly, applicants ask for letters from professors, work supervisors, PAs, nurse practitioners, physicians, volunteer supervisors, or research mentors. Regardless of who you ask, it is of the utmost importance that the writer knows you well enough to write a strong letter. They should be able to attest to attributes such as your academic prowess, clinical experience, work with patients, interpersonal skills, perseverance, dedication, motivation, intelligence, scientific aptitude, reliability, and ability to work as part of a team in the letter. Remember that a weak or mediocre letter of recommendation can be a red flag for admissions committees, so choose people who you are confident will write you great letters. Of note, it is also important to choose people who are reliable and timely. You should provide your letter writers with at least one month of advanced notice so that they have ample time to compose your letter and submit it through CASPA or other application avenues by the appropriate deadline.

Links for Further Information

- Central Application Service for Physician Assistants: https://portal.caspaonline.org/caspaHelpPages/about-caspaoverview/index.html
- Physician Assistant Education Association Program Directory: www.directory.paeaonline.org

PROGRAM ATTRIBUTES

Overview

Here we provide key information that helps to distinguish programs from one other and to help you narrow down your list of programs. For each program we provide the mission statement, curriculum structure, PANCE scores, and unique program features (if available).

Mission Statement

Each PA program has a mission statement that in addition to stating that it wants to produce well-trained PAs, also includes other specific attributes that can tune applicants into the focus of the program and whether or not they might be a good fit for that program. Let's examine some examples:

> *The mission of the Yale School of Medicine Physician Associate Program is to educate individuals to become outstanding clinicians and to foster leaders who will serve their communities and advance the physician assistant profession.*

> *The Physician Assistant Studies Program at the University of South Dakota provides a comprehensive primary care education that prepares graduates to deliver high quality healthcare to meet the needs of patients in South Dakota and the region.*

> *The mission of the Child Health Associate/Physician Assistant Program at the University of Colorado is to provide comprehensive physician assistant education in primary care across the lifespan, with expanded training in pediatrics and care of the medically underserved.*

Though each of the above statements is short, they tell us important attributes about the programs and the types of students that they are trying to recruit. The PA Program at Yale, in addition to creating well-trained PAs, wants to foster leaders that will serve the community and advance the profession. Applicants with aspirations to eventually obtain local or national leadership roles, or with significant amounts of leadership experience in their undergraduate training, prior employment, or volunteer work may align best with the mission statement of Yale and may have a better chance of acceptance than those without leadership aspirations or experience. The PA Program at the University of South Dakota emphasizes primary care in their mission statement, as well as creating providers who will care for patients in South Dakota and the surrounding areas. Thus, applicants with ties to South Dakota and the surrounding states, as well as interest in pursuing a career in primary care will likely have increased chances of admission compared to those who plan to practice in other areas of the country or in different specialties. Finally, the program at the University of Colorado focuses on pediatrics and care of the medically underserved. If you have an interest in pursuing a career in pediatrics, or have prior experience caring for medically underserved populations, you might be a good fit for this program. These examples emphasize the importance of understanding the mission of each PA program and choosing programs that align with your career goals and prior experience to increase your chances of acceptance and to find the perfect program for you.

Curriculum Structure

The curriculum structure of each program can vary significantly. In general, programs can be divided into three different phases: the didactic phase, the clinical phase, and the graduate project phase.

Didactic Phase

The first phase is the didactic phase. During this phase, students complete the majority of their coursework, learn to take a history and perform a physical exam, learn basic clinical skills, and are introduced to the clinical world through different patient encounters and experiences. The didactic phase generally ranges from 10-24 months, with most programs ranging from 12-16 months. Within the didactic phase, there are several types of teaching methodologies that are implemented. These also vary by program with some programs focusing on one modality and others having more of a mixed-methods approach. Some methods that programs utilize include lectures, discussion, case-based learning, team-based learning, inquiry-based learning, small group work, projects, self-guided learning, clinical skills workshops, and others. We provide for you the duration of the didactic phase, and encourage you to learn about the different types of teaching methods that each program employs (and what they mean) by visiting the program website and asking questions during the interview process.

Clinical Phase

The second phase is the clinical phase of the program, which is primarily focused on clinical exposure and skills development. It is meant to solidify and employ the information obtained from the didactic phase through interactions with real patients. It generally consists of a series of clinical rotations, interspersed with "call-back days" where students return to campus to take rotation specific examinations, listen to lectures on various topics about PA practice and clinical medicine, and participate in workshops. The clinical phase typically ranges from 12-18 months. Each rotation itself can range from 2-12 weeks, with most rotations ranging from 4-8 weeks depending on the program. Generally, programs with longer rotations or shorter clinical phases have fewer elective rotations built in for students. We have provided the number of required and elective rotations, as well as the duration of each rotation for each school.

Graduate Project Phase

The third phase of most PA programs is the graduate project phase. Since most programs offer Masters degrees, most programs have built in some type of Masters requirement. In some programs, this is a Capstone Project that students must complete within the local community. Other programs require students to complete a literature review on a topic of interest or to complete a research thesis project. There are also some programs that do not require a graduate project at all, though this is becoming less common. For each program, we have included the type of project required, if any, as part of the curriculum and graduation requirements.

PANCE Scores

The PANCE passing rates for each program are an important metric for applicants, as PAs must pass the PANCE in order to be certified and ultimately practice as a PA. A student who completes an accredited program but does not pass the PANCE is not able to practice. Furthermore, the first-time pass rates (the percentage of students who pass the PANCE on the first attempt) are of the utmost importance because the chances of passing the PANCE decrease with each attempt, and because the PANCE is an expensive test, currently costing $475. Of course, the PANCE is also a metric of the knowledge obtained in PA school and thus how well a program has prepared a PA student to be a PA. We have provided the first-time PANCE pass rates for each program for both the most recent year, as well as cumulative pass rates over the last 5 years. The average PANCE pass rate each year ranges from 90-95%.

Unique Program Features

In this section we provide the distinguishing features, unique opportunities, and interesting aspects of each program that students can use to differentiate programs and as talking points during the interview process. This information is gathered both from program websites as well as from the perspectives of currently enrolled students to provide applicants with the most up-to-date information about each program. Example program features include things such as availability of international rotations, new facilities, medical mission trips, dual degree options, research opportunities, and community service experiences among others.

PA PROGRAM DATA 2015

200
total accredited
PA programs

65% private,
33% public,
2% either both
public/private or
military

65%
private
57%
non-profit,
8%
for profit

67%
located
at a non-academic
medical center

33%
located at an
academic medical
center

Average Program
length: **27 months**

93%
offer a Master's degree
(all required by 2020)

Average tuition
non-resident:
$75,964;
resident
$64,961

Average student to
faculty ratio:
13:1

Top 3 reasons students
choose a PA program:

(1) Conversation with
program faculty

(2) Program reputation

(3) Program location

Average class size
44.5 students per
year and a total of
approximately 8200
first year students
nationally

Average GPA of
Matriculating Students:
3.52 (science 3.47 and
non-science 3.54)

Average GPA of
Applicants:
3.34 overall,
3.46 non-science,
3.24 science

Average GRE Percentile: Math **50%,** Verbal **42%,** Analytical **48%**

Gender of Matriculants: **70.3%** female, **29.7%** male

Average age at matriculation: **26**

Average age at application: **26**

94% of PA programs participate in CASPA

22,997 unique applicants and **190,721** overall applications for 2015

Average number of programs applied to: **8.3**

Average cost of application: **$490**

Top 4 Majors of Matriculants: Biology, Psychology, Chemistry, Health Sciences

Healthcare experience average: **4177 hours** of direct patient care and 1343 of other related experience

Programs requiring supplemental application: **60%**

Average supplemental application fee: **$53**

Median new graduate salary: **$86,000**

CASPA Opening Date: **April 27, 2016**

ALABAMA

UNIVERSITY OF ALABAMA AT BIRMINGHAM

University of Alabama at Birmingham

430 School of Health Professions

1705 University Boulevard
Birmingham, AL 35244
Phone: 205-934-3209
Email: Askcds@uab.edu

Mission: The mission of the UAB Physician Assistant Program is to provide qualified individuals with the knowledge, skills, and judgment needed to assist physicians in the care of patients in surgical and medical settings.

Accreditation:
Continued

Degree Offered:
Master (MSPAS)

Start Date:
August annually

Program Length:
27 months

Class Capacity:
90 students

Tuition: In-state:
$59,735; Out-of-state:
Approximately $120,000

GPA Requirement:
Overall GPA 3.0;
Science GPA 3.0;
Prerequisite GPA 3.0

Healthcare Experience:
500 hours required

PA Shadowing:
Preferred, not required

Required Standardized Testing: GRE or MCAT

Letters of Recommendation:
Three required; no one specific

Seat Deposit: $300

CASPA Participant: Yes

Supplemental Application: Yes

Admissions: Not specified

Application Deadline:
September 1

Class of 2017
Male: 21%
Female: 79%
Minority: 29%
GPA: 3.54
Science GPA: 3.47
GRE Verbal:
58th percentile
GRE Quantitative:
46th percentile
GRE Writing:
not reported
Faculty to Student Ratio: not reported
Average Healthcare Experience:
3,446 hours

PANCE Scores
5-year First Time Pass:
98%
Most Recent First Time Pass: 100%

Curriculum Structure
Didactic: 15 months
Clinical: 12 months
Rotations:
7 mandatory, 5 electives;
4 weeks each
Master's Research Project Presentation:
Required for graduation

Prerequisite Coursework

Biology I and II with lab preferred (6-8 credits), Microbiology with lab preferred (3-4 credits), Human Anatomy and Physiology (6-8 credits), General Chemistry with lab preferred (8-9 credits), Statistics with lab preferred (3-4 credits), Psychology (6 credits).

Unique Program Features

Surgical Focus: While the program prepares students to pass PANCE, it has a surgical focus with cadaveric dissections, coursework in surgical diseases, surgical technique, operating room technique, simulation training, and up to five elective rotations in surgical settings.

Admissions Preference: Approximately 50% of students in the Class of 2017 were Alabama residents, while the other 50% came from other states.

Class of 2017

Male: 35%
Female: 65%
Minority: not reported
GPA: 3.62
Science GPA: 3.60
GREVerbal: 155
GRE Quantitative: 154
GRE Writing: 4.0
Faculty to Student Ratio: not reported
Average Healthcare Experience: 1,845 hours

PANCE Scores

5-year First Time Pass: 92%

Most Recent First Time Pass: 88%

Curriculum Structure

Didactic: 15 months
Clinical: 12 months
Rotations: 7 mandatory, 2 electives; 4-8 weeks each
Capstone Project: Required for graduation

UNIVERSITY OF SOUTH ALABAMA

University of South Alabama

5721 USA Drive North
HAHN 3124
Mobile, AL 36688
Phone: 251-445-9334
Email: pastudies@southalabama.edu

Mission: The mission of the University of South Alabama Physician Assistant Program is to educate compassionate and competent individuals from diverse backgrounds to become highly qualified physician assistants in accordance with the highest professional standards to provide a broad spectrum of preventative and curative healthcare to patients in various communities and clinical settings with physician supervision including underserved populations in Alabama both rural and urban. The emphasis of the program is one of primary care, including a broad foundation in the medical and surgical specialties.

Accreditation: Continued

Degree Offered: Master (MHS)

Start Date: May annually

Program Length: 27 months

Class Capacity: 40 students

Tuition: In-state: $50,336; Out-of-state: $100,672

GPA Requirement: Overall GPA 3.0

Healthcare Experience: 500 hours required

PA Shadowing: Not required

Required Standardized Testing: GRE (minimum of 145 on verbal and quantitative and 3.5 on writing)

Letters of Recommendation: Three required; one letter from a MD/DO/PA

Seat Deposit: $500

CASPA Participant: Yes

Supplemental Application: Yes

Admissions: Not specified

Application Deadline: November 1

Prerequisite Coursework

Biology (3 credits), General Chemistry I and II with lab (8 credits), Organic Chemistry or Biochemistry (3 credits), General Microbiology (3 credits), Human Anatomy and Physiology (6 credits), Mathematics (3 credits), Statistics (3 credits), General Psychology (3 credits), Medical Terminology (2 credits). Courses may be in progress at time of application as long as they are completed prior to the start of the program. Students will be given bonus points in the admissions process if they have taken genetics, biochemistry, immunology, physics, pathophysiology or pharmacology coursework.

Unique Program Features

Primary Care Focus:
The program has a focus on primary care and you can read about student experiences on the primary care rotation on their website.

Admissions Preference:
There is a preference for Alabama applicants, but the program will consider applicants from all states. The program is also dedicated to recruiting veterans and saves up to 10 seats per class for qualified veterans.

Community Service:
Students are committed to community health outreach and offered free health screenings for diabetes, breast cancer, hypertension, and STDs as well as education regarding drugs, alcohol, skin cancer, vaccines, diet, and exercise. You can read about community services and other program happenings in the news section of their website.

ARIZONA

ARIZONA SCHOOL OF HEALTH SCIENCES

Arizona School of Health Sciences

5850 E. Still Circle
Mesa, AZ 85206
Phone: 480-219-6030
Email: btrahan@atsu.edu

Mission: The A.T. Still University Department of Physician Assistant Studies provides a learning-centered education that develops exemplary physician assistants who deliver whole person healthcare with an emphasis on underserved populations.

Accreditation: Continued

Degree Offered: Master (MSPAS)

Start Date: June annually

Program Length: 26 months

Class Capacity: 70 students

Tuition: $75,486

GPA Requirement: Overall GPA 2.75; Science GPA 2.75.

Healthcare Experience: Encouraged, not required.

PA Shadowing: Not required.

Required Standardized Testing: N/A

Letters of Recommendation: Three required; (1) Employer or supervisor (2) Health Care Practitioner (Physician, Physician Assistant or Nurse Practitioner), and (3) Science Faculty Member.

Seat Deposit: $1500

CASPA Participant: Yes

Supplemental Application: Yes

Admissions: Rolling

Application Deadline: September 1

Class of 2016

Male: not reported
Female: not reported
Minority: not reported
GPA: 3.56
Prerequisite GPA: 3.50
GRE: not required
Faculty to Student Ratio: not reported
Average Healthcare Experience: not reported

PANCE Scores

5-year First Time Pass: 91%

Most Recent First Time Pass: 96%

Curriculum Structure

Didactic: 14 months
Clinical: 12 months
Rotations: 7 mandatory, 1 elective rotation; 6 weeks in duration.
Capstone Paper/Project: Required for graduation

Prerequisite Coursework

Human Anatomy with lab, Human Physiology with lab, Microbiology, Biochemistry, College Algebra or Statistics, Medical Terminology (1-3 credits). Anatomy, Physiology and Microbiology are recommended to be completed within 5 years of the application date. Prerequisites may be in progress at time of application.

Unique Program Features

Hometown Scholars Program: This program promotes the provision of high-quality, comprehensive healthcare that is accessible, coordinated, culturally and linguistically competent and community-directed for all underserved populations for applicants interesting in pursuing community health. Typically applicants work or volunteer in a community health center and then obtain an endorsement from the community health center leadership which is used as part of the application process.

Class of 2017

Male: 30%
Female: 70%
Minority: not reported
GPA: 3.68
Science GPA: 3.64
GREVerbal: 71st percentile
GRE Quantitative: 66th percentile
GRE Writing: 4.4 (70th percentile)
Faculty to Student Ratio: not reported
Average Healthcare Experience: not reported

PANCE Scores

5-year First Time Pass: 98%

Most Recent First Time Pass: 99%

Curriculum Structure

Didactic: 13.5 months
Clinical: 13.5 months
Rotations: 7 mandatory, 2 elective rotation; 6 weeks in duration.

Master's Portfolio: Required for graduation

MIDWESTERN UNIVERSITY (GLENDALE)

Midwestern University
Email: admissaz@midwestern.edu

19555 59th Avenue
Glendale, AZ 85254
Phone: 623-572-3614

Mission: The Midwestern University Physician Assistant Program is committed to educate and mentor students in a setting that cultivates excellence and prepares compassionate, competent physician assistants to serve in a changing healthcare environment.

Accreditation: Continued

Degree Offered: Master (MMS)

Start Date: June annually

Program Length: 27 months

Class Capacity: 90 students

Tuition: $94,667

GPA Requirement: Overall GPA 2.75; Science GPA 2.75; Prerequisite GPA 2.75.

Healthcare Experience: Preferred, not required.

PA Shadowing: Not required.

Required Standardized Testing: GRE

Letters of Recommendation: Two required; no one specific.

Seat Deposit: $750

CASPA Participant: Yes

Supplemental Application: No

Admissions: Rolling

Application Deadline: October 1

Prerequisite Coursework

Biology with lab (8 credits), General Chemistry with lab (8 credits), Organic Chemistry with lab (4 credits), Math (3 credits), English Composition (6 credits), Social and Behavioral Sciences (6 credits). Biochemistry and Statistics are recommended. Prerequisites can be in progress at time of application.

Unique Program Features

Inter-professional Education: Every first-year PA student participates in a university wide inter-professional course that serves to highlight commonalities between the professions. Program faculty and students also participate in several inter-professional community service opportunities that include providing medical care to the medically underserved communities in the Phoenix area.

NORTHERN ARIZONA UNIVERSITY

Northern Arizona University
NAU Graduate College

PO Box 4125
Flagstaff, AZ 86011
Phone: 602-827-2450
Email: PAProg@nau.edu

Mission: The mission of the Northern Arizona University Physician Assistant Studies Program is to recruit individuals of the highest possible quality from diverse backgrounds and life experiences to the profession and to equip them with clinical and professional knowledge, skills and abilities to provide high quality, compassionate medical care for the people of Arizona.

Accreditation:
Provisional

Degree Offered:
Master (MPAS)

Start Date:
August annually

Program Length:
24 months

Class Capacity:
50 students

Tuition:
In-state: $29,474;
Out-of-state: $56,332

GPA Requirement:
Overall GPA 3.0;
Science GPA 3.0;

Healthcare Experience:
500 hours minimum

PA Shadowing:
Not required.

Required Standardized Testing: GRE

Letters of Recommendation: Three required; no one specific. Email addresses must be provided to the program.

Seat Deposit: $0

CASPA Participant: Yes

Supplemental Application: Yes

Admissions:
Rolling

Application Deadline:
September 1

Prerequisite Coursework

Chemistry (2 courses), Anatomy, Physiology, Statistics, Microbiology, 1 Hands-on Lab course, Upper Division Science (4 courses). 9 credits of science must be taken in the past five years, and 40 credits of sciences overall must be completed. All courses must be completed at the time of application.

Class of 2016
Male: not reported
Female: not reported
Minority: not reported
GPA: 3.5
Science GPA: 3.5
GREVerbal: not reported
GRE Quantitative: not reported
GRE Writing: not reported
Faculty to Student Ratio: not reported
Average Healthcare Experience: not reported

PANCE Scores
5-year First Time Pass: 96% (based on two years of data)
Most Recent First Time Pass: 96%

Curriculum Structure
Didactic: 12months
Clinical: 12months
Rotations:
7 mandatory, 2 selectives in primary care, 2 elective rotations; 4 weeks in duration.
Capstone Project: Required for graduation

Unique Program Features

Medical School Partnership: The program is a collaboration between Northern Arizona University and The University of Arizona College of Medicine – Phoenix which enhances the student experience with access to world-class lecturers, up-to-date technology, simulation centers and inter-professional education.

State Sponsored School: This is the only state school PA program in Arizona and recruits students from Arizona as well as those with ties to the region who plan to practice in Arizona in the future, particularly in rural and underserved areas.

ARKANSAS

HARDING UNIVERSITY

Harding University
Email: paprogram
@harding.edu

915 E. Market
HU 12231
Searcy, AR 72149
Phone: 501-279-5642

Mission: Developing caring physician assistants who practice competent, patient-centered primary care in diverse environments.

Accreditation:
Continued

Degree Offered:
Master (MSPAS)

Start Date:
August annually

Program Length:
28 months

Class Capacity:
36 students

Tuition:
$79,000

GPA Requirement:
Overall GPA 3.0;
Prerequisite GPA 3.0

Healthcare Experience:
100 hours required

PA Shadowing:
Not required

Required Standardized Testing: GRE

Letters of Recommendation: Three required; no one specific

Seat Deposit: $300

CASPA Participant: Yes

Supplemental Application: Yes

Admissions: Not specified

Application Deadline:
November 1

Prerequisite Coursework

General Chemistry I and II with labs (8 credits), Organic Chemistry or Biochemistry (3 credits), Microbiology with lab (4 credits), Human Anatomy with lab (4 credits), Human Physiology with lab (4 credits), College Algebra or Calclulus or Statistics (3 credits), General or Developmental Psychology (3 credits), Psychology elective (3 credits), Upper Level Biology (3 credits). Only 1 prerequisite course may be left for completion during the spring semester (winter quarter) prior to the program start date the following fall.

Unique Program Features

Medical Terminology: Students must pass a medical terminology exam at the interview to be considered for acceptance in the program.

Christian Faith: The University has strong Christian values and teaches physician assistants who practice within a framework of dependence on God and faith.

Class of 2016

Male: not reported
Female: not reported
Minority:
not reported
GPA: 3.59
Prerequisite GPA:
3.64
GRE: not required
Faculty to Student Ratio: not reported
Average Healthcare Experience: 1,786

PANCE Scores

5-year First Time Pass:
93%

Most Recent First Time Pass: 100%

Curriculum Structure

Didactic: 12 months
Clinical: 16 months
Rotations: 7 mandatory, 1 electives, 1 preceptorship; 6 weeks each
Master's Project: required for graduation

Class of 2017

Male: 24%
Female: 76%
Minority: 15%
GPA: 3.59
Science GPA: 3.46
GRE: 308 (verbal and quantitative)
Faculty to Student Ratio: not reported
Average Healthcare Experience: 2,712

PANCE Scores

5-year First Time Pass: N/A

Most Recent First Time Pass: N/A (have not graduated a class yet)

Curriculum Structure

Didactic: 13 months
Clinical: 15 months
Rotations: 10 mandatory, 2 electives; 3-5 weeks each
Capstone Project: required for graduation

Unique Program Features

Service Learning: The didactic phase includes a required service learning component across the lifespan of geriatrics, pediatrics, and adults. This is approximately 10 hours per semester.

Facilities: The program has state-of-the-art facilities including lecture halls, small group space, physical exam laboratory, clinical skills laboratory, and a simulation center.

University of Arkansas

4301 W. Markham Slot 772
Little Rock, AR 72205
Phone: 501-686-7211
Email: paprogram@gmail.com

Mission: The mission of the UAMS Physician Assistant Program is to educate students who will practice patient-centered medicine while embracing cultural diversity, ethical integrity, professionalism and collaboration with other members of the health care team. The program fosters lifelong learning through emphasis on critical thinking, clinical application of knowledge and evidence-based medicine. Through innovative educational practices, the students will be prepared to enter into any discipline of medicine with the ability to serve any community and contribute to the profession through leadership, education, and service.

Accreditation: Provisional

Degree Offered: Master (MPAS)

Start Date: May annually

Program Length: 28 months

Class Capacity: 38 students

Tuition:
In-state: $42,000;
Out-of-state: $70,000

GPA Requirement: None (Overall GPA and Science GPA of 3.0 are recommended)

Healthcare Experience: 500 hours required

PA Shadowing: Recommended, not required

Required Standardized Testing: GRE

Letters of Recommendation: Three required; one from a physician or PA, one from a university/college professor, one from a supervisor.

Seat Deposit: $300

CASPA Participant: Yes

Supplemental Application: Yes

Admissions: Not specified

Application Deadline: November 1

Prerequisite Coursework

General Biology I and II with lab (8 credits), Human Anatomy with lab (4 credits), Human Physiology with lab (4 credits), Microbiology with lab (4 credits), Medical Genetics (3 credits), General Chemistry I and II with lab (8 credits), Organic Chemistry I with lab (4 credits), General Psychology (3 credits), Abnormal Psychology (3 credits), Biostatistics or Statistics (3 credits. Anatomy, Physiology and Microbiology must be completed in the last seven years. Up to two in progress prerequisites are allowed at time of application.

CALIFORNIA

LOMA LINDA UNIVERSITY

Loma Linda University
Email: pa@llu.edu

24785 Stewart Street
Evans Hall 201
Loma Linda, CA 92350
Phone: 909-558-7295

Mission: The Loma Linda University Department of Physician Assistant Sciences educates primary care physician assistants who will complement the work of physicians by providing health care as active members of a professional healthcare team, excellence and compassion in health care for the whole person, and quality health care for underserved individuals and communities nationally and globally in accordance with the mission of Loma Linda University and the School of Allied Health Professions.

Accreditation:
Continuing

Degree Offered:
Master (MPA)

Start Date:
September annually

Program Length:
24 months

Class Capacity:
36 students

Tuition:
$82,500

Seat Deposit: $500

GPA Requirement:
Overall GPA 3.0;
Science GPA 3.0

Healthcare Experience:
2,000 hours required

PA Shadowing:
Not required

Required Standardized Testing: None

Letters of Recommendation: Three required; one letter must be from a currently practicing physician, DO or PA with whom the applicant has worked in a paid patient care position.

CASPA Participant: Yes

Supplemental Application: Yes

Admissions: Not specified

Application Deadline:
October 1

Class of 2017
Male: 47%
Female: 53%
Minority: not reported
GPA: 3.53
Science GPA: not reported
GRE: not required
Faculty to Student Ratio: not reported
Average Healthcare Experience: not reported

PANCE Scores
5-year First Time Pass: 94%
Most Recent First Time Pass: 94%

Curriculum Structure
Didactic: 12 months
Clinical: 12 months
Rotations: 7 mandatory, 1 electives; 6 weeks each
Capstone Project: required for graduation

Prerequisite Coursework

Human Anatomy and Physiology with lab (8 credits), General Chemistry with lab or a sequence in Inorganic, Organic, and Biochemistry with lab (8 credits), General Microbiology with lab (4 credits), General Psychology, General Sociology or Cultural Anthropology, College-level Algebra or equivalent, English (1 year). A maximum of 2 total prerequisite courses be outstanding at the time of application, with only 1 science prerequisite outstanding.

Unique Program Features

Primary Care Focus:
This program has a primary care focus and specifically a focus on caring for the underserved.

Medical Spanish:
Students are required to take a medical Spanish course and participate in a local Spanish immersion program. Students are split into tracks according to proficiency levels.

International Rotations: Currently the program has rotation sites in Honduras and Malawi with more sites in development.

Admissions Preference: The program gives preference to Seventh-day Adventists, graduates of Loma Linda, applicants of under-represented populations, and applicants with a history of meaningful, continuous involvement in community service.

MARSHALL B. KETCHUM UNIVERSITY

Marshall B. Ketchum University
Email:
PAadmissions@ketchum.edu

2575 Yorba Linda Boulevard
Fullerton, CA 92831
Phone: 714-992-7808

Mission: Our Mission is to educate individuals to become compassionate physician assistants who can provide the highest quality health care, are dedicated to their communities, and practice evidence-based medicine while promoting population health and advancing the Physician Assistant profession.

Accreditation:
Provisional

Degree Offered:
Master (MMS)

Start Date:
August annually

Program Length:
27 months

Class Capacity:
40 students

Tuition: $93,700

Seat Deposit: $1,500

GPA Requirement:
Overall GPA 3.0;
Science GPA 3.0

Healthcare Experience:
1,000 hours required

PA Shadowing:
Not required

Required Standardized Testing: None

Letters of Recommendation:
Three required; one from a professor, one from an immediate supervisor, and one from a health professional.

CASPA Participant: Yes

Supplemental Application: Yes

Admissions: Non-rolling

Application Deadline:
November 1

Prerequisite Coursework

Biological Sciences (16 credits) which must include Microbiology with lab, Human Anatomy with lab, and Human Physiology with lab. Biochemistry or Organic Chemistry (3 credits), Statistics (3 credits), General Psychology (3 credits). Human Anatomy and Physiology should be completed within the last 10 years and all courses must be completed at the time of application.

Unique Program Features

Medical Spanish: An elective in medical Spanish is available for interested students.

Inter-professional Education: PA students in Marshall B. Ketchum interact with Optometry and Pharmacy students throughout the curriculum in working on clinical cases and completing coursework in ethics.

Integrated Curriculum: Integration of curricula in medical education seeks to break down barriers between subject areas in order to provide students with better learning opportunities that will facilitate the development of knowledge.

PANCE Scores

5-year First Time Pass: 95%

Most Recent First Time Pass: 96%

Curriculum Structure

Didactic: 15 months

Clinical: 12 months

Rotations: 7 mandatory, 2 electives; 4 weeks each

Unique Program Features

Medical Simulation: The program makes extensive use of high fidelity medical simulation technology and manikins throughout the didactic and clinical curriculum.

International Rotations: International rotations are available to students as are rotations where students can participate in community health with underserved patients in the San Francisco Bay Area.

SAMUEL MERRITT UNIVERSITY

Samuel Merritt University
Email: admission@samuelmerritt.edu

3100 Telegraph Avenue
Suite 1000
Oakland, CA 94609
Phone: 510-869-6576

Mission: The Master Physician Assistant Department at Samuel Merritt University strives to serve the University and the medical community by preparing graduates who are interdependent medical providers, demonstrate commitment to the community and the profession through active leadership, manifest critical and creative thinking, utilize effective communication skills, and who possess the educational foundation for continued growth and development in a changing world of diverse cultures.

Accreditation: Continued

Degree Offered: Master (MPA)

Start Date: September annually

Program Length: 27 months

Class Capacity: 44 students

Tuition: $91,464

GPA Requirement: Overall GPA 3.0; Science GPA 3.0

Healthcare Experience: 1,000 hours recommended

PA Shadowing: Not required

Required Standardized Testing: None

Letters of Recommendation: Three required; two from health care professionals who have supervised or worked with you and one academic letter

Seat Deposit: $350

CASPA Participant: Yes

Supplemental Application: No

Admissions: Non-rolling

Application Deadline: October 1

Prerequisite Coursework

Biological Sciences (16 credits) which must include Microbiology with lab, Human Anatomy with lab, and Human Physiology with lab, Statistics (3 credits), Inorganic/General Chemistry (4 credits), Organic Chemistry or General Chemistry II (4 credits). Preference is given to those who have completed courses in the last 5 years.

STANFORD UNIVERSITY

Stanford University

Phone:
650-725-6959

1215 Welch Road
Modular G
Palo Alto, CA 94305-5408
Email: pcap-information@lists.stanford.edu

Mission: The mission of the Primary Care Associate Program is: to educate PAs for clinical practice in primary care and medically underserved communities in California;to increase the enrollment and deployment of under-represented minorities; and to respond to the needs of our communities and stakeholders, including Stanford Medical Center.

Accreditation:
Continued

Degree Offered:
Associate (AS),
Master (MMS)

Start Date:
June annually

Program Length:
21 months

Class Capacity:
50 students

Tuition:
$52,094

GPA Requirement:
Science GPA 3.0;
Prerequisite GPA 2.0

Healthcare Experience:
3,000 hours required

PA Shadowing:
Not required

Required Standardized Testing: None

Letters of Recommendation: Three required; one from a physician, one from a PA, and one from a clinical supervisor

Seat Deposit: $400

CASPA Participant: No
Supplemental Application: No

Admissions: Non-rolling
Application Deadline:
October 1

Class of 2016 and 2017

Male: 37%
Female: 63%
Minority: 38%
GPA: not reported
Science GPA: not reported
GRE: not required
Faculty to Student Ratio: not reported
Average Healthcare Experience: 8,792 hours

PANCE Scores

5-year First Time Pass: 89%

Most Recent First Time Pass: 91%

Curriculum Structure

Didactic: 9 months
Clinical: 12 months
Rotations: Students are placed with a preceptor from their home community for several months of primary care and then are placed in emergency medicine, inpatient care, surgery, and long-term care rotations.

Prerequisite Coursework

Human Anatomy with lab (4 credits), Human Physiology with lab (4 credits), Microbiology with lab (4 credits), General Chemistry (3 credits), Intermediate Algebra (3 credits), English Composition (3 credits), Introduction to Sociology or Introduction to Cultural Anthropology (3 credits), Introduction to or General Psychology (3 credits). Grades for all courses must be completed by the application deadline October 1. It is recommended that Anatomy, Physiology and Microbiology be completed within the last five years.

Unique Program Features

Primary Care Focus:
This program has a focus on primary care, placing students in primary care rotations within their home communities. 58% of graduates go on to practice in primary care settings.

Master of Medical Sciences: The MMS degree is completed through an articulation agreement online with St.

Francis University during the course of the PA program. Students take four additional courses.

Community Satellites:
The program is recruiting students from current target communities including Kern County, Humboldt County, Imperial County, Salinas area, San Diego County, and the Ventura/Los Angeles area.

Class of 2017

Male: 20%

Female: 80%

Minority: 45%

GPA: 3.22

Science GPA: 3.17

GRE: not required

Faculty to Student Ratio: not reported

Average Healthcare Experience: not reported

PANCE Scores

5-year First Time Pass: 98%

Most Recent First Time Pass: 100%

Curriculum Structure

Didactic: 16.5 months

Clinical: 16.5 months (including MPH fieldwork)

Rotations: 6 mandatory, 2 elective; 6 weeks each

MPH Capstone: required for graduation

TOURO UNIVERSITY - CALIFORNIA

Touro University

1310 Club Drive
Vallejo, CA 94592
Phone: 707-638-5200
Email: tucpa@tu.edu

Mission: Through the integration of the Physician Assistant and Public Health disciplines, the mission of the Joint MSPAS/MPH Program is to: 1) train quality PAs to work with underserved populations, 2) recruit applicants from these communities or individuals with a demonstrated interest in serving these communities, and 3) increase access to care for underserved populations

Accreditation: Continued

Degree Offered: Master (MSPAS, MPH)

Start Date: August annually

Program Length: 33 months

Class Capacity: 44 students

Tuition: $119,800

GPA Requirement: Overall GPA 2.75; Science GPA 2.75;

Healthcare Experience: 500 hours required

PA Shadowing: 20 hours or more preferred

Required Standardized Testing: None

Letters of Recommendation: Three required; one from a clinician and two general non-family letters

Seat Deposit: $400

CASPA Participant: Yes

Supplemental Application: Yes

Admissions: Not specified

Application Deadline: November 1

Unique Program Features

Dual Degree: All students complete a dual MSPAS/MPH degree program integrating clinical medicine and population health. This is the only program that mandates a dual degree for all PA students.

Admissions Preference: Proficiency in Spanish or other foreign languages in considered an advantage for the applicant in the admissions process.

Prerequisite Coursework

Biological Sciences with lab (8 credits), Chemistry with lab (8 credits), Human Anatomy with lab (4 credits), Human Physiology with lab (4 credits), Microbiology with lab (4 credits), Statistics (3 credits). Anatomy and Physiology must be completed within 5 years of expected matriculation and all courses must be completed at the time of application.

UNIVERSITY OF CALIFORNIA-DAVIS

University of California-Davis

4610 X Street Suite 4202
Sacramento, CA 95817
Phone: 916-734-2145
Email: BettyIreneMooreSON
@ucdmc.ucdavis.edu

Mission: The mission of the Family Nurse Practitioner and Physician Assistant Program (FNP/PA) is to educate health care professionals to deliver care as a member of a health care team and to improve the availability of culturally relevant primary health care in underserved populations throughout California.

Accreditation:
Continued

Degree Offered:
Master (MHS)

Start Date:
June annually

Program Length:
27 months

Class Capacity:
40 students

Tuition:
$114,302

GPA Requirement:
Overall GPA 3.0;
Science GPA 2.75;

Healthcare Experience:
1000 hours required

PA Shadowing:
Not required

Required Standardized Testing: None

Letters of Recommendation: Three required; no one specific

Seat Deposit: not specified

CASPA Participant: Yes

Supplemental Application: Yes

Admissions: Non-rolling

Application Deadline:
July 15

No class statistics reported

PANCE Scores
5-year First Time Pass: 97%

Most Recent First Time Pass: 92%

Curriculum Structure
Didactic: 12 months

Clinical: 15 months

Rotations:
7 mandatory, no information on electives or duration

Master's Thesis:
required for graduation

Prerequisite Coursework

Human Anatomy with lab, Human Physiology with lab, General Chemistry with lab, Microbiology or Bacteriology with lab, Algebra or Calculus or Statistics, English Composition, Social Sciences (two courses). All must be completed at the time of application.

Unique Program Features

Inter-professional Education: This is the only program that combines both PA and nurse practitioner students in the same classroom for the didactic curriculum and includes both the medical school model and nursing model of education blended throughout.

Primary Care Focus: The program focuses on primary care and 60% of graduates work in underserved areas while 59% of graduates work in primary care.

Class of 2017 and 2018

Male: 25%
Female: 75%
Minority: 60%
GPA: 3.49
Science GPA: 3.41
GRE: 307
MCAT: 27
Faculty to Student Ratio: not reported
Average Healthcare Experience: 2,585 hours

PANCE Scores

5-year First Time Pass: 96%
Most Recent First Time Pass: 95%

Curriculum Structure

Didactic: 12 months preclinical, 4 months post clinical, one summer off
Clinical: 12 months
Rotations: 8 mandatory, 1 elective, no duration reported

UNIVERSITY OF SOUTHERN CALIFORNIA

University of Southern California

Email: uscpa@usc.edu

1000 S. Fremont Avenue
Unit 7, Building A-11, Room 150
Alhambra, CA 91803
Phone: 626-457-4240

Mission: The Primary Care Physician Assistant Program at USC is dedicated to the advancement of physician assistant education and emphasizes service to the medically underserved. The program is committed to preparing students from diverse backgrounds to practice medicine with physician supervision. Emphasis is placed upon understanding and appreciating diversity. The program aims to prepare its graduates to practice and promote primary health care of the highest quality as part of an inter-professional team

Accreditation: Continued

Degree Offered: Master (MPAP)

Start Date: August annually

Program Length: 33 months

Class Capacity: 60 students

Tuition: $148,392

GPA Requirement: Overall GPA 3.0; Science GPA 2.75; Prerequisite GPA 3.0

Healthcare Experience: Preferred, not required

PA Shadowing: Preferred, not required

Required Standardized Testing: GRE or MCAT

Letters of Recommendation: Three required; no one specific

Seat Deposit: $500

CASPA Participant: Yes
Supplemental Application: Yes

Admissions: Rolling
Application Deadline: November 1

Unique Program Features

Leadership: The program aims to train PA leaders and has been successful as graduates have gone on to become members of Congress, President of AAPA and CAPA, as well as various other roles in national and local organizations.

Advocacy Education: Students receive training in advocacy through the Medical Care Organization course and Advanced Topics in Education. Students also volunteer for a program trip to Washington, DC where attendees learn how to advocate for the profession from the AAPA and PAEA staff.

Community Service: Students serve the homeless and underserved populations of Los Angeles through student run clinics, food drives, and other initiatives.

Prerequisite Coursework

General Biology I and II with lab, General Chemistry I and II with lab, Human Anatomy with lab (3 credits), Human Physiology with lab (3 credits), General Microbiology with lab (3 credits), Statistics (3 credits), Introduction to Psychology (3 credits), Spanish (2 semesters), English Composition (2 semesters for international applicants only). All sciences courses must be completed within 10 years of application deadline and must be completed by the end of the fall semester prior to matriculation.

WESTERN UNIVERSITY OF HEALTH SCIENCES

Western University of Health Sciences

Email:
Admissions@westernu.edu

309 E. Second Street
Pomona, CA 91766
Phone: 909-469-5378

Mission: The Department of Physician Assistant Education supports the University's mission by educating Physician Assistants to deliver high quality competent and compassionate health care as team members within the health care delivery system.

Accreditation:
Continued

Degree Offered:
Master (MSPA)

Start Date:
August annually

Program Length:
24 months

Class Capacity:
98 students

Tuition: $76,930

GPA Requirement:
Overall GPA 2.7;
Science GPA 2.7;
Prerequisite GPA 2.7

Healthcare Experience:
Preferred, not required

PA Shadowing: Preferred, not required

Required Standardized Testing: None

Letters of Recommendation: Two required; no one specific

Seat Deposit: $500

CASPA Participant: Yes

Supplemental Application: Yes

Admissions: Not specified

Application Deadline:
November 1

Class of 2017

Male: not reported
Female: not reported
Minority: not reported
GPA: 3.57
Science GPA: 3.57
Prerequisite GPA: 3.67
GRE: not required
Faculty to Student Ratio: not reported
Average Healthcare Experience: not reported

PANCE Scores

5-year First Time Pass: 91%

Most Recent First Time Pass: 97%

Curriculum Structure

Didactic: 12 months

Clinical: 12 months

Rotations:
8 mandatory, electives and duration not reported

Master's Thesis:
Required for graduation

Prerequisite Coursework

English Composition (6 credits), College Algebra (3 credits), Human Anatomy and Physiology with lab (6 credits), Microbiology with lab, Genetics, Psychology, Sociology, introductory Statistics, General or Inorganic Chemistry with lab (6 credits), Humanities (9 credits). All courses must be completed by spring semester prior to matriculation and no more than one science and non-science prerequisite can be in progress after December 31.

Unique Program Features

Inter-professional Education: PA students complete case studies with Osteopathic Medicine, PA, Physical Therapy, Pharmacy, Nursing, Veterinary, Optometry and Dental students during their didactic curriculum.

Student Experiences: You can read about student experiences in the program on the website under the section entitled "Testimonials".

COLORADO

RED ROCKS COMMUNITY COLLEGE

Red Rocks Community College

Email: pa.program@rrcc.edu

13300 W. 6th Avenue

Lakewood, CO 80228

Phone: 303-914-6386

Mission: The mission of the Red Rocks Community College Physician Assistant program is to train clinically competent and compassionate physician assistants to provide primary care to the medically underserved.

Accreditation: Continued

Degree Offered: Master (MPAS)

Start Date: August annually

Program Length: 27 months

Class Capacity: 32 students

Tuition: In-state: $37,584; Out-of-state: $45,868

GPA Requirement: None

Healthcare Experience: 2,000 hours required

PA Shadowing: Not required

Required Standardized Testing: none

Letters of Recommendation: Three required; no one specific

Seat Deposit: $500

CASPA Participant: Yes

Supplemental Application: Yes

Admissions: Not specified

Application Deadline: August 1

Class of 2017

Male: 28%
Female: 72%
Minority: not reported
GPA: 3.31
Science GPA: not reported
GRE: not required
Faculty to Student Ratio: not reported
Average Healthcare Experience: not reported

PANCE Scores

5-year First Time Pass: 94%

Most Recent First Time Pass: 94%

Curriculum Structure

Didactic: 13 months
Clinical: 14 months
Rotations: 11 mandatory, 1 elective, 1 preceptorship, 4 weeks each
Capstone Project: required for graduation

Prerequisite Coursework

College Algebra or higher (3 credits), Statistics (3 credits), Physics (3 credits), Cell Biology or Genetics (3 credits), Additional Biology (9 credits), Organic Chemistry (3 credits), Additional Chemistry (7 credits). All courses must be completed by June 15 of the year you apply.

Unique Program Features

Curriculum Sequence: Students complete two didactic semesters, then complete three primary care rotations, followed by another didactic semester before finishing the balance of the clinical curriculum. This allows students to put into practice knowledge early in their training.

Problem Based Learning: In addition to traditional lecture formal, problem based learning is integrated into every semester of the program, including clinical rotations when students meet for call back days.

Primary Care Focus: The College has collaborated with Colorado Counties Incorporated, Colorado Municipal League, and the Special Districts Association which together make up the Colorado Collaboration for Rural Healthcare Access with the goal of increasing the primary care and rural workforce in Colorado.

Class of 2018

Male: 20%

Female: 80%

Minority: 16%

GPA: 3.69

Science GPA: 3.64

GRE Verbal: 73rd percentile

GRE Quantitative: 62nd percentile

GRE Analytical: not reported

Faculty to Student Ratio: not reported

Average Healthcare Experience: 2,087 hours

PANCE Scores

5-year First Time Pass: 98%

Most Recent First Time Pass: 98%

Curriculum Structure

Didactic: 18 months

Clinical: 18 months

Rotations: vary based on track

Capstone Project: required for graduation

University of Colorado
Email:
pa-info@ucdenver.edu

13001 E. 17th Place
Mail Stop F543
Aurora, CO 80045
Phone: 303-724-7963

Mission: The mission of the Child Health Associate/Physician Assistant Program is to provide comprehensive physician assistant education in primary care across the lifespan, with expanded training in pediatrics and care of the medically underserved.

Accreditation: Continued

Degree Offered: Master (MPAS)

Start Date: June annually

Program Length: 36 months

Class Capacity: 44 students

Tuition:
In-state: $47,838;
Out-of-state: $103,582

GPA Requirement:
Overall GPA 2.8;
Science GPA 2.8

Healthcare Experience: Preferred, not required

PA Shadowing: Not required

Required Standardized Testing: GRE

Letters of Recommendation: Three required; no one specific

Seat Deposit: $1,065

CASPA Participant: Yes

Supplemental Application: Yes

Admissions: Rolling

Application Deadline: September 1

Unique Program Features

Specialized Tracks: The program offers specialized tracks in rural medicine, global health, urban/underserved medicine, LEADS (leadership, education, advocacy, development, and scholarship), and pediatric critical and acute care.

Pediatrics Focus: Though the program prepares PAs to care for patients of all ages, students complete at least 3 dedicated pediatrics rotations in addition to other rotations such as family medicine which incorporates the pediatric population.

Profiles: The program provides profiles of selected current students, graduates, and preceptors to get a feel for the students accepted into the program, the outcomes for graduates, and the preceptors that students will interact with in clinical rotations.

Prerequisite Coursework

Chemistry (8 credits), Biology (14 credits which must include 1 semester of Anatomy and 1 semester of Physiology), General Genetics (3 credits), Psychology (6 credits), Statistics (3 credits). The Chemistry and Biology requirements must be completed prior to application.

CONNECTICUT

QUINNIPIAC UNIVERSITY

Quinnipiac University

Physician Assistant Program

370 Bassett Road
North Haven, CT 06473
Phone: 203-582-8672
Email: paadmissions@quinnipiac.edu

Mission: The mission of Quinnipiac's physician assistant program is to increase access to quality health care through the education and development of caring, knowledgeable and competent physician assistants who are dedicated to clinical competence, professionalism, leadership, community outreach, and cultural competence.

Accreditation:
Continued

Degree Offered:
Master (MHS)

Start Date:
May annually

Program Length:
27 months

Class Capacity:
54 students

Tuition:
$87,022

Seat Deposit: $500

GPA Requirement: Overall GPA 3.0, cumulative science GPA 3.0. The most competitive applicants should possess an overall GPA of 3.2 and cumulative science GPA of 3.2.

Healthcare Experience: The most competitive applicants should possess at a minimum 2,500 hours of direct patient care experience in the U.S. healthcare system.

PA Shadowing: Not required

Required Standardized Testing: None

Letters of Recommendation: two required

CASPA Participant: Yes

Supplemental Application: No

Admissions: Not rolling

Application Deadline:
September 1

Class of 2015
Male: 32%
Female: 68%
Minority: 8%
GPA: 3.56
Science GPA: 3.55
GRE: not required
Faculty to Student Ratio: not reported
Average Healthcare Experience:
3,000 hours

PANCE Scores

5-year First Time Pass: 98%

Most Recent First Time Pass: 100%

Curriculum Structure

Didactic: 15 months (12 months to start, and 3 months to end the program)

Clinical: 12 months

Rotations:
7 mandatory, 2 elective rotations; each mandatory rotation is 6 weeks while each elective is 4 weeks

Capstone Project:
Part of graduation requirement

Prerequisite Coursework

4 semesters of biology with labs to include at least one semester of microbiology and 2 semesters of anatomy and physiology

3 semesters of chemistry with

labs to include at least one semester of biochemistry or organic chemistry

Pre-calculus or Calculus or Statistics

*Applicant can have maximum of two prerequisites in progress at time of application and all must be completed by Dec 31

Unique Program Features

Community Service:
Students are very active in the local community with mandatory service completed throughout the program. They have made the largest contribution to the AAPA Host City Prevention Campaign each of the last 12 years.

Facilities:
The program is housed within the brand new medical building of the Frank Netter School of Medicine which features 24 teaching labs, cadaver dissection lab, simulation rooms, 16 standardized patient rooms, multiple team study rooms, and expanded health science library, and a student lounge.

Urban Health Scholars Program:
18 students in 2014 participated in this program which is a collaboration between the University of Connecticut and the Connecticut Area Health Education Center to provide primary care and health literacy education to urban communities in the state.

UNIVERSITY OF BRIDGEPORT

University of Bridgeport
Physician Assistant Institute
Email: PAI@bridgeport.edu

126 Park Ave.
Bridgeport, CT 06604
Phone: 203-576-2400

Mission: The mission of the University of Bridgeport Physician Assistant Institute is to develop clinicians with: dedication to patients; commitment to life-long education; respect for the profession; a global perspective on health care; volunteerism as a professional core value and integrative approach to practice for the benefit of all patients. The motto is: Adiuvare (to help), Mederi (to heal), Communiter (together).

Accreditation:
Administrative Probation

Degree Offered:
Master (MS)

Start Date:
January annually

Program Length:
28 months

Class Capacity:
40 students

Tuition:
$90,650

Seat Deposit: $750

GPA Requirement:
3.0 overall GPA;
3.0 science GPA

Healthcare Experience: 500 hours of direction patient care experience required.

PA Shadowing: not required

Required Standardized Testing: None

Letters of Recommendation:
Three required; one must be from a healthcare provider and another from a supervisor of the clinical experience. The third can be a professor, employer, or another individual who has known the applicant on a professional level for a year or more.

CASPA Participant: Yes

Supplemental Application: Yes

Admissions: Rolling

Application Deadline:
August 1

PANCE Scores
5-year First Time Pass: 84%

Most Recent First Time Pass: 98%

Curriculum Structure
Didactic: 14 months
Clinical: 14 months (6 weeks of which are summative testing and cumulative review at the end of the program)
Rotations: 7 mandatory, 1 elective rotation, each 6 weeks long.
CapstoneProject: required as a part of graduation requirements.

Prerequisite Coursework

Anatomy and Physiology, Biology, General Chemistry I and II, English, Psychology, Statistics, Microbiology, Genetics, Biochemistry

Unique Program Features

Integrative Medicine: Students complete coursework in complementary and alternative medicine throughout the didactic curriculum which includes topics such as chiropractic medicine, acupuncture, and naturopathy to gain perspective as to how these professionals may be beneficial to their future patients.

Global Health: The curriculum interweaves global health into many courses, culminating with a Global Health course in the last didactic semester which offers the student the opportunity to investigate the impact of health issues in other countries and the interactive effect on all populations in terms of epidemiology, disease, disasters, economics, health initiatives, ethics and policy

YALE UNIVERSITY

Yale School of Medicine Physician Associate Program
Email: pa.program@yale.edu

100 Church Street South, A250
PO Box 208083
New Haven, CT 06520
Phone: 203-785-2860

Mission: The mission of the Yale School of Medicine Physician Associate Program is to educate individuals to become outstanding clinicians and to foster leaders who will serve their communities and advance the physician assistant profession.

Accreditation: Continued

Degree Offered: Master (MMSc)

Start Date: August annually

Program Length: 28 months

Class Capacity: 45 students

Tuition: $83,162

GPA Requirement: Science GPA 3.0

Healthcare Experience: 1,000 hours recommended, not required

PA Shadowing: Recommended, not required

Required Standardized Testing: GRE

Letters of Recommendation: Three required; one from a healthcare professional and two others of the applicant's choice.

Seat Deposit: $1,000

CASPA Participant: Yes

Supplemental Application: Yes

Admissions: Rolling

Application Deadline: October 1

Prerequisite Coursework

Statistics or Calculus, Human Anatomy, Human or Animal Physiology, Organic or Biochemistry, Microbiology, Genetics. One prerequisite may be in progress upon applying and must be completed by December 31.

Unique Program Features

International Rotations: Students can utilize an elective rotation to study abroad at pre-approved sites throughout Europe, Asia, Africa, and South America.

Dual Degree Option: Students can apply to both the PA program and public health school at the same time. If accepted to both, students complete a dual MPH/MMSc degree program of 39 months duration.

Research: Student complete a research project proposal as a requirement for graduation and have an integrated research course including journal clubs throughout the didactic year.

Surgical Anatomy: Students complete a full-cadaver dissection using surgical cases as a guide to optimize applicability of acquired skills to the operating room setting and clinical practice

DISTRICT OF COLUMBIA

GEORGE WASHINGTON UNIVERSITY

George Washington
University
Email:
paadm@gwu.edu

2100 Pennsylvania Avenue, NW
3rd Floor, Suite 300
Washington, DC 20037
Phone: 202-994-7644

Mission: The George Washington University Physician Assistant Program educates Physician Assistant students to practice evidence-based medicine, advocate for patients, and serve their communities.

Accreditation:
Continuing

Degree Offered:
Master (MSHS)

Start Date:
June annually

Program Length:
24 months

Class Capacity:
68 students

Tuition: $83,640

GPA Requirement:
Overall GPA: 3.0;
Science GPA: 3.0;
Prerequisite GPA 2.75

Healthcare Experience:
1,000 hours required

PA Shadowing:
Not required

Required Standardized Testing: GRE

Letters of Recommendation: Two required; no one specific

Seat Deposit: $1,000

CASPA Participant: Yes

Supplemental Application: Yes

Admissions: Not specified

Application Deadline:
October 1

Prerequisite Coursework

Anatomy, Physiology, Chemistry (2 semesters, one must be either Organic Chemistry or Biochemistry), Psychology, Statistics. Courses must be completed with a "B-" or better within the last 10 years.

Unique Program Features

Dual Degree: Students can complete a 3 year dual MPH/MSHS degree in one of three specialty tracks including Community Oriented Primary Care, Health Policy, and Epidemiology.

Student Society: The Tolton Society is very active in helping students obtain leadership roles, service activities, and establishing a National Medical Challenge Bowl team to compete at the annual PA conference. In addition, students are encouraged to participate in professional advocacy and many descend upon Capitol Hill to discuss issues confronting the PA profession with congressional representatives.

PANCE Scores

5-year First Time Pass: 86%

Most Recent First Time Pass: 96%

Curriculum Structure

Didactic: 16 months

Clinical: 12 months

Rotations: Information not provided

Unique Program Features

Admissions: The program focuses on providing a PA educational opportunity to promising Black students and other ethnically diverse minority students.

HOWARD UNIVERSITY

Howard University
Email:
paadmissions@howard.edu

516 Bryant Street NW, #119
Annex 2
Washington, DC 20059
Phone: 202-806-7536

Mission: The mission of the Howard University Physician Assistant Program is to recruit and prepare compassionate and competent physician assistants with expertise in clinical decision-making, problem solving, and research for the enhancement of the health of the public and the advancement of the profession on local, national, and international levels.

Accreditation: Continuing

Degree Offered: Master (MPAS)

Start Date: August annually

Program Length: 28 months

Class Capacity: 35 students

Tuition: $64,350

GPA Requirement: Overall GPA: 3.0; Science GPA: 3.0; Prerequisite GPA 3.0

Healthcare Experience: 200 hours required for Master's applicants

PA Shadowing: Not required

Required Standardized Testing: GRE

Letters of Recommendation: Three required; no one specific

Seat Deposit: None

CASPA Participant: Yes

Supplemental Application: Yes

Admissions: Not specified

Application Deadline: January 15

Prerequisite Coursework

English Composition (2 semesters), Algebra I and II, Intro to Sociology, Biology, Microbiology with lab, Intro to Psychology, Chemistry I and II with lab, Community Health, Technical Writing, Medical Terminology, Computer Technology, Nutrition. These are the courses that the entry-level students must complete before moving onto the Master's curriculum.

FLORIDA

ADVENTIST UNIVERSITY OF HEALTH SCIENCES

Adventist University of
Health Sciences
Email: pa.info@adu.edu

671 Winyah Drive
Orlando, FL 32803
Phone: 407-303-8778

Mission: Our program seeks to educate individuals in becoming knowledgeable, compassionate and spiritually uplifting healthcare providers. Whether they practice locally, nationally, or globally, the PA program graduates individuals who embrace a mission of service to others

Accreditation:
Provisional

Degree Offered:
Master (MSPAS)

Start Date:
May annually

Program Length:
27 months

Class Capacity:
25 students

Tuition:
$60,000

Seat Deposit: $500

GPA Requirement:
Overall GPA 3.0;
Science GPA 3.0

Healthcare Experience:
2000 hours recommended, not required

PA Shadowing: Preferred, not required

Required Standardized Testing: GRE

Letters of Recommendation:
Three required; at least one recommendation must arrive from a practicing physician assistant or physician. No more than one letter may come from a professor.

CASPA Participant: Yes

Supplemental Application: No

Admissions: Not specified

Application Deadline:
October 1

Prerequisite Coursework

General Chemistry I and II (8 credits), Organic Chemistry I and II (8 credits), Biochemistry I and II (7 credits), Anatomy and Physiology I and II (8 credits), General Biology I and II (8 credits), General Microbiology (4 credits), English Composition I and II (6 credits), Medical Terminology (2 credits), General Psychology (3 credits), Developmental Psychology (3 credits), Abnormal Psychology (3 credits), Elementary Statistics (3 credits). Science courses should be current within 7 years of program matriculation.

Class of 2017
Male: not reported
Female: not reported
Minority:
not reported
GPA: 3.36
Science GPA: not reported
GRE: not reported
Faculty to Student Ratio: not reported
Average Healthcare Experience: not reported

PANCE Scores
5-year First Time Pass:
N/A

Most Recent First Time Pass: N/A (have not graduated a class yet)

Curriculum Structure
Didactic: 15 months
Clinical: 12 months
Rotations:
7 mandatory, 2 elective; 4 weeks each.
Capstone Project:
Required for graduation

Unique Program Features
Medical Missions: Students in good standing can participate in a medical mission field project that will be arranged through the University during the clinical year.

Facilities: There is a newly renovated PA lab with 11 fully outfitted patient examination bays where students learn to take histories, perform physical exams, and learn clinical procedures.

PANCE Scores

5-year First Time Pass: 91%

Most Recent First Time Pass: 90%

Curriculum Structure

Didactic: 16 months (12 preclinical and 4 post-clinical)

Clinical: 12 months

Rotations: 7 mandatory, 1 elective; 6 weeks each.

Library Research Paper: Required for graduation

Unique Program Features

One Program, Three Locations: The program utilizes innovative technology to conduct instructional education via interactive video conferencing. Live lecturers present at one of three locations in Miami, St. Croix, or St. Petersburg. Students in the locations without the live lecturer are connected via the video conferencing.

Medical Spanish: All students complete a 40 hours total immersion Medical Spanish course.

BARRY UNIVERSITY

Barry University
Email:
paadmissions@barry.edu

11300 NE 2nd Avenue
Miami, FL 33161
Phone: 305-899-3293

Mission: The Barry University Physician Assistant Program educates students in practice of collaborative medicine and encourages life-long learning and professional development. It fosters a technology rich environment and clinical training experiences among diverse patient populations. The Program enables students to develop competencies required to meet the health care needs of contemporary society.

Accreditation: Continued

Degree Offered: Master (MCMSc)

Start Date: August annually

Program Length: 28 months

Class Capacity: 52 students (Miami), 24 students (St. Croix), 24 students (St. Petersburg)

Tuition: $76,533

GPA Requirement: Overall GPA 3.0; Science GPA 3.0

Healthcare Experience: Recommended, not required

PA Shadowing: Not required

Required Standardized Testing: GRE

Letters of Recommendation: Three required; no one specific

Seat Deposit: $1000

CASPA Participant: Yes

Supplemental Application: No

Admissions: Rolling

Application Deadline: December 1

Prerequisite Coursework

Biological Sciences (12 credits), Behavioral or Social Sciences (6 credits), General Chemistry (6 credits), Organic Chemistry or Biochemistry (3 credits). Courses must be completed within the last 10 years and up to three can be in progress at time of application.

FLORIDA INTERNATIONAL UNIVERSITY HERBERT WERTHEIM COLLEGE OF MEDICINE

Herbert Wertheim
College of Medicine

Email:
jpomares@fiu.edu

11200 SW 8th Street
MARC Building #260
Miami, FL 33199
Phone: 305-348-6567

Mission: The mission of Florida International University Herbert Wertheim College of Medicine Master in Physician Assistant Studies is to prepare a diverse workforce of masters-level primary care physician assistants to collaboratively practice with physicians and other members of the health care team

Accreditation:
Provisional

Degree Offered:
Master (MPAS)

Start Date:
July annually

Program Length:
27 months

Class Capacity:
45 students

Tuition:
In-state: $53,000;
Out-of-state:
$71,550

Seat Deposit:
$450

GPA Requirement:
Overall GPA 3.0; Science GPA 3.0;
Upper Division GPA 3.0

Healthcare Experience:
Recommended, not required

PA Shadowing: Not required, but applicants with > 300 hours receive additional preference.

Required Standardized Testing: GRE (scores > 152 in each section preferred)

Letters of Recommendation:
Three required; letters should be from Physicians, Physician Assistants, Nurse Practitioners, Professors or any individual who has worked with the applicant in a professional or educational environment.

CASPA Participant: Yes
Supplemental Application: Yes

Admissions: Rolling
Application Deadline:
December 1

Prerequisite Coursework

Mathematics (3 credits), Statistics (3 credits), English (6 credits), Humanities/Art (3 credits), Social Sciences (9 credits), Medical Terminology (1 credit), General Chemistry I and II with lab (8 credits), General Biology I and lab or Zoology and lab (4 credits), General Microbiology (4 credits), Human Anatomy and Physiology with lab (8 credits), Organic Chemistry I with lab (4 credits), Organic Chemistry II with lab or Biochemistry with lab (4 credits), Genetics (3 credits). All courses must be completed by the fall semester in which you apply.

No class statistics reported

PANCE Scores
5-year First Time Pass: N/A

Most Recent First Time Pass: N/A (have not graduated a class yet)

Curriculum Structure
Didactic: 15 months

Clinical: 12 months

Rotations:
8 mandatory,
1 elective;
4-8 weeks each.

Signature Paper:
Required for graduation

Unique Program Features

Pre-Entrance Exam:
Applicants must complete a score Pre-Entrance Exam comprising multiple-choice and essay questions (topics will be provided one month prior to the exam date).

Green Family Foundation NeighborhoodHELP: Students participate in Green Family Foundation NeighborhoodHELP™, HWCOM's signature, longitudinal service learning program, incorporating the social determinants of health. This program provides MPAS students the opportunity to work in inter-professional teams that include medical, nursing, and social work students. These inter-professional teams work directly with underserved households in South Florida, and MPAS students glean hands on experience in providing population based and culturally competent health care.

No class statistics reported

PANCE Scores

5-year First Time Pass: 84% (three years of available data)

Most Recent First Time Pass: 95%

Curriculum Structure

Didactic: 12 months

Clinical: 12 months

Rotations: 7 mandatory, 2 elective; 5 weeks each.

Graduate Project: Required for graduation

Unique Program Features

Not specified

Keiser University
Email: None provided

1500 NW 49th Street
Fort Lauderdale, FL 33309
Phone: 954-776-4456

Mission: The Keiser University physician assistant program provides an environment that fosters quality academic and clinical education. The program, in collaboration with the community, provides physician assistants who excel in integrative patient care, education and service to benefit the public. The program promotes lifelong responsibility for ongoing learning and active participation in a changing healthcare environment.

Accreditation: Provisional

Degree Offered: Master (MSPA)

Start Date: January annually

Program Length: 24 months

Class Capacity: 40 students

Tuition: $66,000

Seat Deposit: $1000

GPA Requirement: Overall GPA 2.75; Science GPA 3.0; Prerequisite GPA 3.0

Healthcare Experience: Recommended, not required

PA Shadowing: Required

Required Standardized Testing: GRE (minimum score of 294)

Letters of Recommendation: Three required; one written by a Physician Assistant, one from a practicing health care provider, and one personal reference

CASPA Participant: Yes

Supplemental Application: Yes

Admissions: Rolling

Application Deadline: November 1

Prerequisite Coursework

College Math (3 credits), English (6 credits), Humanities (3 credits), Social Sciences (3 credits), Behavioral Sciences (6 credits), General Biology or Zoology with lab (4 credits), General Chemistry I and II with lab (8 credits), Microbiology with lab (4 credits), Biochemistry or Organic Chemistry, Human Anatomy and Physiology I and II with labs (8 credits), Genetics (3 credits). Natural Science courses must have been completed in the last 10 years and up to 2 prerequisites can be in progress at time of application.

NOVA SOUTHEASTERN UNIVERSITY – FORT LAUDERDALE

Nova Southeastern University
Enrollment and Processing Services - PA Admissions

3301 College Avenue, PO Box 29900
Fort Lauderdale, FL 33329-9905
Phone: 954-262-1250
Email: dickman@nova.edu

Mission: To provide a primary care training program designed for, and dedicated to, producing competent physician assistants who will provide quality health care in rural, urban, underserved, and culturally diverse communities; to increase the accessibility of quality health care in the primary care setting; to prepare students for lifelong learning and leadership roles; and to promote the physician assistant profession.

Accreditation: Continued

Degree Offered: Master (MMS)

Start Date: June annually

Program Length: 27 months

Class Capacity: 75 students

Tuition: $69,806

CASPA Participant: Yes

Supplemental Application: Yes

Admissions: Not specified

Application Deadline: December 1

GPA Requirement: Overall GPA 3.0; Science GPA 3.0

Healthcare Experience: Recommended, not required

PA Shadowing: Not specified

Required Standardized Testing: GRE

Letters of Recommendation: Three required; one letter of recommendation/evaluation must be sent from an individual (other than a relative or friend) such as an academic advisor, professor, coworker, or supervisor. Two letters of recommendation/evaluation must be from health care professionals, one of which must be from a physician or a PA with whom you have worked, shadowed, or volunteered.

Seat Deposit: $1,000

No class statistics reported

PANCE Scores
5-year First Time Pass: 98%

Most Recent First Time Pass: 99%

Curriculum Structure
Didactic: 15 months
Clinical: 12 months
Rotations: 6 mandatory, 3 elective; 4-6 weeks each.
Graduate Project: Required for graduation

Unique Program Features
Dual Degree Program: Students in any of Nova's PA programs can complete a dual degree MMS/MPH program by simultaneously taking only MPH courses during the PA program. Students typically finish the MPH shortly after the MMS.

Prerequisite Coursework
College Math (3 credits), English (6 credits), Humanities/Arts (3 credits), Social Sciences (9 credits), General Inorganic Chemistry I and II with lab (8 credits), Microbiology with lab (4 credits), General Biology or Zoology with lab (4 credits), Human Anatomy and Physiology (6 credits), Biochemistry or Organic Chemistry (3 credits), Human Genetics (3 credits), Medical Terminology (1 credit). Science prerequisites must be completed by the end of the fall semester prior to matriculation. The remaining prerequisites must be completed by the time of matriculation.

PANCE Scores

5-year First Time Pass: 94%

Most Recent First Time Pass: 96%

Curriculum Structure

Didactic: 14.5 months

Clinical: 12.5 months

Rotations: 6 mandatory, 3 elective; 4-6 weeks each.

Graduate Project: Required for graduation

Unique Program Features

Dual Degree Program: Students in any of Nova's PA programs can complete a dual degree MMS/MPH program by simultaneously taking only MPH courses during the PA program. Students typically finish the MPH shortly after the MMS.

NOVA SOUTHEASTERN UNIVERSITY — FORT MYERS

Nova Southeastern University
Email: jkeena@nova.edu

3650 Colonial Court
Fort Myers, FL 33913
Phone: 239-274-1020

Mission: The NSU Physician Assistant Program - Fort Myers endeavors to provide an exemplary educational experience that emphasizes primary medical care, and enables graduates to demonstrate competency and skill in a variety of clinical environments; prepare students for the pursuit of lifelong learning; prepare students for leadership roles, enabling them to focus on improving access to health care; promote the physician assistant profession.

Accreditation: Continued

Degree Offered: Master (MMS)

Start Date: June annually

Program Length: 27 months

Class Capacity: 60 students

Tuition: $69,806

CASPA Participant: Yes

Supplemental Application: Yes

Admissions: Not specified

Application Deadline: December 1

GPA Requirement: Overall GPA 3.0; Science GPA 3.0

Healthcare Experience: Recommended, not required

PA Shadowing: Not specified

Required Standardized Testing: GRE

Letters of Recommendation: Three required; one letter of recommendation/evaluation must be sent from an individual (other than a relative or friend) such as an academic advisor, professor, coworker, or supervisor. Two letters of recommendation/evaluation must be from health care professionals, one of which must be from a physician or a PA with whom you have worked, shadowed, or volunteered.

Seat Deposit: $1,000

Prerequisite Coursework

College Math (3 credits), English (6 credits), Humanities/Arts (3 credits), Social Sciences (9 credits), General Inorganic Chemistry I and II with lab (8 credits), Microbiology with lab (4 credits), General Biology or Zoology with lab (4 credits), Human Anatomy and Physiology (6 credits), Biochemistry or Organic Chemistry (3 credits), Human Genetics (3 credits), Medical Terminology (1 credit). Science prerequisites must be completed by the end of the fall semester prior to matriculation. The remaining prerequisites must be completed by the time of matriculation.

NOVA SOUTHEASTERN UNIVERSITY – JACKSONVILLE

Nova Southeastern University
Email: cahinfo@nova.edu

6675 Corporate Center Parkway
Suite 115
Jacksonville, FL 32216
Phone: 904-245-8990

PANCE Scores
5-year First Time Pass: 89%
Most Recent First Time Pass: 92%

Mission: To provide an exemplary educational experience, which emphasizes primary medical care, yet will enable graduates to manifest competency and skill in a variety of clinical environments. To inspire graduates to pursue lifelong learning. To foster leadership qualities, which will enable graduates to improve access to quality, affordable health care. To heighten the stature of the physician assistant profession.

Curriculum Structure
Didactic: 14 months
Clinical: 13 months
Rotations: 6 mandatory, 3 elective; 4-6 weeks each.
Graduate Project: Required for graduation

GPA Requirement: Overall GPA 3.0; Science GPA 3.0

Healthcare Experience: Recommended, not required

PA Shadowing: Not specified

Required Standardized Testing: GRE

Letters of Recommendation: Three required; one letter of recommendation/evaluation must be sent from an individual (other than a relative or friend) such as an academic advisor, professor, coworker, or supervisor. Two letters of recommendation/evaluation must be from health care professionals, one of which must be from a physician or a PA with whom you have worked, shadowed, or volunteered.

Seat Deposit: $500

Accreditation: Continued

Degree Offered: Master (MMS)

Start Date: June annually

Program Length: 27 months

Class Capacity: 60 students

Tuition: $69,806

Unique Program Features

Dual Degree Program: Students in any of Nova's PA programs can complete a dual degree MMS/MPH program by simultaneously taking only MPH courses during the PA program. Students typically finish the MPH shortly after the MMS.

Prerequisite Coursework

College Math (3 credits), English (6 credits), Humanities/Arts (3 credits), Social Sciences (9 credits), General Inorganic Chemistry I and II with lab (8 credits), Microbiology with lab (4 credits), General Biology or Zoology with lab (4 credits), Human Anatomy and Physiology (6 credits), Biochemistry or Organic Chemistry (3 credits), Human Genetics (3 credits), Medical Terminology (1 credit). Science prerequisites must be completed by the end of the fall semester prior to matriculation. The remaining prerequisites must be completed by the time of matriculation.

CASPA Participant: Yes

Supplemental Application: Yes

Admissions: Not specified

Application Deadline: December 1

PANCE Scores

5-year First Time Pass: 99%

Most Recent First Time Pass: 98%

Curriculum Structure

Didactic: 15 months

Clinical: 12 months

Rotations: 7 mandatory, 1 selective, 1 elective; 4-6 weeks each.

Graduate Project: Required for graduation

Unique Program Features

Dual Degree Program: Students in any of Nova's PA programs can complete a dual degree MMS/MPH program by simultaneously taking only MPH courses during the PA program. Students typically finish the MPH shortly after the MMS.

NOVA SOUTHEASTERN UNIVERSITY — ORLANDO

Nova Southeastern University
Email: cahinfo@nova.edu

6675 Corporate Center Parkway
Suite 115
Jacksonville, FL 32216
Phone: 904-245-8990

Mission: To provide high quality training program designed for and dedicated to producing culturally competent physician assistants who will provide quality health care in rural, urban, underserved, and culturally diverse communities. To provide an exemplary educational experience, which emphasizes primary medical care, yet will enable graduates to manifest competency and skill in a variety of clinical environments. To inspire graduates to pursue lifelong learning. To foster leadership qualities that will enable graduates to improve access to quality and affordable healthcare. To heighten the stature of the physician assistant profession by training quality graduates.

Accreditation: Probation

Degree Offered: Master (MMS)

Start Date: May annually

Program Length: 27 months

Class Capacity: 64 students

Tuition: $69,806

CASPA Participant: Yes

Supplemental Application: Yes

Admissions: Not specified

Application Deadline: January 15

GPA Requirement: Overall GPA 3.0; Science GPA 3.0

Healthcare Experience: Recommended, not required

PA Shadowing: Not specified

Required Standardized Testing: GRE

Letters of Recommendation: Three required; one letter of recommendation/evaluation must be sent from an individual (other than a relative or friend) such as an academic advisor, professor, coworker, or supervisor. Two letters of recommendation/evaluation must be from health care professionals, one of which must be from a physician or a PA with whom you have worked, shadowed, or volunteered.

Seat Deposit: $1,000

Prerequisite Coursework

College Math (3 credits), English (6 credits), Humanities/Arts (3 credits), Social Sciences (9 credits), General Inorganic Chemistry I and II with lab (8 credits), Microbiology with lab (4 credits), General Biology or Zoology with lab (4 credits), Human Anatomy and Physiology (6 credits), Biochemistry or Organic Chemistry (3 credits), Human Genetics (3 credits), Medical Terminology (1 credit). Science prerequisites must be completed by the end of the fall semester prior to matriculation. The remaining prerequisites must be completed by the time of matriculation.

MIAMI-DADE COLLEGE

MDC Medical Campus
Email:
jhernan7@mdc.edu

950 NW 20th St.
Miami, FL 33127
Phone: 305-237-4124

Mission: The mission of the PA program is to (1) Provide high quality education and training opportunities in primary care for students from diverse cultural backgrounds interested in providing health care services to the medically under-served residents in urban and rural communities, especially in Florida; (2) Promote and maintain high academic and professional standards; (3) Participate in professional activities and continuing education to promote life-long learning; (4)Prepare each graduate with a level of didactic and clinical competence that provides successful entry into the profession.

Accreditation:
Continued

Degree Offered:
Associate, optional
Masters (MMS)

Start Date:
August annually

Program Length:
24 months

Class Capacity:
50 students

Tuition:
In-state: $22,188;
Out-of-state: $38,109

GPA Requirement:
General Education GPA 2.5;
Natural Science GPA 2.7;

Healthcare Experience:
Recommended, not required

PA Shadowing: 50 hours
recommended, not required

**Required Standardized
Testing:** None

**Letters of
Recommendation:** Three
required; no one specific

Seat Deposit: Not specified

CASPA Participant: No

**Supplemental
Application:** No

Admissions: Not specified

Application Deadline:
November 15

Prerequisite Coursework

Introduction to Healthcare, English Composition I (3 credits), Fundamentals of Speech Communication (3 credits), The Psychology of Personal Effectiveness (3 credits), Critical Thinking and Ethics (3 credits), Statistical Methods (3 credits), Human Anatomy and Physiology I and II with lab (8 credits), Chemistry for Health Sciences with lab (4 credits), Microbiology with lab (4 credits), Introduction to Microcomputer Usage (1 credit) or Computer Competency Test. All natural science courses taken more than 5 years ago must be repeated.

No class statistics reported

PANCE Scores
5-year First Time Pass: 82%

Most Recent First Time Pass: 91%

Curriculum Structure
Didactic: 12 months
Clinical: 12 months
Rotations:
8 mandatory,
0 elective;
4-8 weeks each.

Unique Program Features

Admissions Test:
Required of applicants who make the initial cut and consists of 100 multiple choice questions in anatomy, physiology, medical terminology, microbiology and math.

Admissions Preference:
This program gives preference to Miami-Dade County residents, however all applicants are considered.

MMS Degree Option:
Though the program awards an Associate's degree, students can complete an online program through St. Francis University to earn the MMS clinical year or shortly thereafter at an additional charge.

Class of 2017

Male: 25%

Female: 75%

Minority: 25%

GPA: 3.4

Science GPA: 3.4

GRE: not reported

Faculty to Student Ratio: not reported

Average Healthcare Experience: 937 hours

PANCE Scores

5-year First Time Pass: 88% (based on four years of data)

Most Recent First Time Pass: 82%

Curriculum Structure

Didactic: 15 months

Clinical: 12 months

Rotations: 7 mandatory, 1 elective; 6 weeks each.

Unique Program Features

Not specified

SOUTH UNIVERSITY – TAMPA

South University, Tampa
Physician Assistant Program
Attention: Admissions Department

4401 North Himes Avenue
Tampa, FL 33614
Phone: 813-393-3720
Email: Not provided

Mission: The Physician Assistant Program at South University - Tampa exists to educate a diverse student population to become providers of high-quality healthcare who will practice the art and science of medicine with physician supervision. The program encourages lifelong learning and research skills with proficiency in critical thinking and problem solving.

Accreditation: Continued

Degree Offered: Master (MSPA)

Start Date: January annually

Program Length: 27 months

Class Capacity: 24 students

Tuition: $68,535

GPA Requirement: Overall GPA 2.8; Science GPA 3.0

Healthcare Experience: Recommended, not required

PA Shadowing: Not specified

Required Standardized Testing: GRE (preference for those with scores > 50th percentile)

Letters of Recommendation: Not specified

Seat Deposit: $500

CASPA Participant: Yes

Supplemental Application: No

Admissions: Not specified

Application Deadline: August 1

Prerequisite Coursework

Human Anatomy (1 semester or quarter), Human Physiology (1 semester or quarter), General Biology (2 semesters or quarters), General Chemistry (2 semesters or quarters), Organic Chemistry (1 semester or quarter), Microbiology (1 semester or quarter), Medical Terminology (1 course).

UNIVERSITY OF FLORIDA

University of Florida
College of Medicine

Email:
admissions@pap.ufl.edu

Box 100176
Gainesville, FL 32610
Phone: 352-265-7955

Mission: The mission of the School of Physician Assistant Studies is to recruit high quality students to become exemplary physician assistants who will serve the people of Florida and the nation as part of a multidisciplinary healthcare team.

Accreditation:
Continued

Degree Offered:
Master (MPAS)

Start Date:
June annually

Program Length:
24 months

Class Capacity:
60 students

Tuition:
In-state: $55,320;
Out-of-state: $122,993

Seat Deposit: $200

CASPA Participant: Yes

Supplemental Application: Yes

Admissions: Not specified

Application Deadline:
September 1

GPA Requirement: None, but successful applicants rarely fall below an Overall GPA of 3.0 and Science GPA of 3.0

Healthcare Experience:
Recommend 2,000 hours, not required

PA Shadowing: Not specified

Required Standardized Testing: GRE (preference for those with scores > 50th percentile)

Letters of Recommendation:
Three required; the School recommends at least one reference from a physician who has supervised the applicant in a clinical setting, one reference from a PA who is familiar with the applicant's clinical work, and one reference from another health professional who has worked alongside the applicant and/or is familiar with the applicant's clinical skills.

Class of 2017
Male: 27%
Female: 73%
Minority: 33%
GPA: 3.5
(range 3.03-3.99)
Science GPA: 3.5
(range 3.01-4.0)
GREVerbal: 155
(range 148-166)
GRE Quantitative:
157 (range 146-161)
GRE Writing:
4.3 (range 3.0-5.0)
Faculty to Student Ratio: not reported
Average Healthcare Experience: 2.3 years (range 0.5 – 10.25 years)

PANCE Scores
5-year First Time Pass: 98%

Most Recent First Time Pass: 99%

Curriculum Structure
Didactic: 12 months
Clinical: 12 months
Rotations:
10 mandatory,
2 elective;
4 weeks each

Prerequisite Coursework

Human Anatomy and Physiology with lab (6-8 credits), Microbiology with lab (3-5 credits), General Chemistry I and II with labs (8-11 credits), Statistics (3 credits), Medical Terminology (1 credit). All courses must have been completed by the fall semester prior to the Program's academic year beginning in late June. Preference is given to applicants whose courses are no older than 5 years.

Unique Program Features

Community Service: Students have several community service opportunities throughout the curriculum. Most notably, students work in student-run, free healthcare clinics that are sponsored by the College of Medicine during their first and second year.

Admissions Preference: This is a state school and each year approximately 80% of students are residents of Florida and 20% come from other states.

GEORGIA

EMORY UNIVERSITY

Emory University
Physician Assistant
Program
Email: not provided

1462 Clifton Rd N.E. Suite 280
Atlanta, GA 30322
Phone: 404-727-7825

Mission: Our mission is to recruit, educate and mentor a diverse group of students to become highly regarded, sought after physician assistants providing compassionate health care of the highest quality. To that end we create an educational environment that promotes an understanding of human needs and ethical issues as well as the acquisition and application of patient-oriented clinical knowledge and skills.

Accreditation:
Continuing

Degree Offered:
Master (MMSc)

Start Date:
August annually

Program Length:
29 months

Class Capacity:
54 students

Tuition:
$100,092

GPA Requirement:
Overall GPA: 3.0;
Science GPA: 3.0;

Healthcare Experience:
2000 hours

PA Shadowing:
Recommended

Required Standardized Testing: GRE (preferred: Verbal 153; Quantitative 144; Analytical Writing 4.0).

Letters of Recommendation: Two required; no one specific

Seat Deposit: $1,000

CASPA Participant: Yes
Supplemental Application: Yes

Admissions: Rolling
Application Deadline: October 1

Prerequisite Coursework

Biology with lab (4 credits), General Chemistry with lab (8 credits), Human Anatomy and Physiology with lab (8 credits), Organic or Biochemistry (3 credits), Statistics or Biostatistics (3 credits). Courses should be completed by December of the application year.

Unique Program Features

Dual Degree: Emory offers a dual degree MPH/MMSc program through the Rollins School of Public Health which typically takes just over 3 years to complete.

Student Information: The website offers student-specific pages for each class so prospective applicants can learn about the happenings in the program with each class.

Senior Mentoring Project: First year students form relationships with seniors in the community to learn more about geriatric medicine and life for older patients. PA students work with medical and nursing students in this endeavor.

Class of 2017

Male: 12%
Female: 88%
Minority: not reported
GPA: 3.50
Science GPA: 3.40
GRE Total: 308
Faculty to Student Ratio: not reported
Average Healthcare Experience: 2,911 hours

PANCE Scores

5-year First Time Pass: 94%

Most Recent First Time Pass: 98%

Curriculum Structure

Didactic: 13 months
Clinical: 15 months
Rotations: 9 mandatory, 2 elective, 5 weeks each
Capstone Project: Required for graduation

MERCER UNIVERSITY

Mercer University
Email: paprogram@mercer.edu

3001 Mercer University Drive
AACC Building, Room 447
Atlanta, GA 30341
Phone: 678-547-6391

Mission: The mission of the Mercer University Physician Assistant Program is to educate patient-centered medical providers of the highest quality who are leaders and life-long learners, possess an appreciation of ethical values and human diversity, and are provided a foundation to practice in every discipline of allopathic medicine. The Physician Assistant Program emphasizes evidence-based medicine, informatics, critical decision making, interdisciplinary teamwork, and continuous quality improvement.

Accreditation: Continuing
Degree Offered: Master (MMSc)
Start Date: January annually
Program Length: 28 months
Class Capacity: 50 students
Tuition: $72,184

CASPA Participant: Yes
Supplemental Application: Yes
Admissions: Not specified
Application Deadline: March 1

GPA Requirement:
Overall GPA: 3.0;
Science GPA: 2.9;
Prerequisite GPA: 2.9
Healthcare Experience: 1000 hours
PA Shadowing: Recommended
Required Standardized Testing: GRE (Combined score of 300 and Analytical score of 3.5 required).
Letters of Recommendation: Three required; one from a practicing PA, MD, or DO, one froma College-Level Instructor, and one from a Non-Relative
Seat Deposit: $1,000

Prerequisite Coursework

General Chemistry I and II with lab, Organic Chemistry, Biochemistry, General Biology I and II with lab, Human Anatomy and Physiology I and II with lab, Microbiology with lab, English Composition or intensive writing (2 courses), Statistics or Biostatistics, General or Introductory Psychology. Anatomy and Physiology should be completed within 10 years of enrollment to PA program.

Unique Program Features

Godsey-Matthews Student Society: The society is very active and was awarded the Outstanding Silver Student Society Award by SAAAPA in 2014 and the Outstanding Bronze Student Society Award in 2012.

Good Samaritan Health Clinic: Didactic and clinical Mercer PA students partner with faculty and other healthcare providers to extend medical care to the underinsured and uninsured patients in the community.

Medical Mission Trips: Students have recently traveled to Haiti, Nicaragua, and Ecuador to deliver healthcare.

SOUTH UNIVERSITY

South University
Email:
paprogram
@southuniversity.edu

709 Mall Boulevard
Savannah, GA 31406
Phone: 912-201-8171

Mission: The South University, Savannah Physician Assistant Studies program exists to educate a diverse student population as providers of high quality, cost-efficient health care who will make a positive difference while practicing the art and science of medicine with physician direction.

Accreditation:
Continuing

Degree Offered:
Master (MSPA)

Start Date:
January annually

Program Length:
27 months

Class Capacity:
70 students

Tuition: $71,280

GPA Requirement:
Overall GPA: 3.0;

Healthcare Experience:
Recommended, not required

PA Shadowing:
Not required

Required Standardized Testing: GRE

Letters of Recommendation:
Three required; one from a physician, DO, PA-C, or NP

Seat Deposit: $500

CASPA Participant: Yes

Supplemental Application: No

Admissions: Not specified

Application Deadline:
August 1

Prerequisite Coursework

Human Anatomy, Human Physiology, General Biology I and II, General Chemistry I and II, Biochemistry or Organic Chemistry, Microbiology.

PANCE Scores

5-year First Time Pass: 95%

Most Recent First Time Pass: 90%

Curriculum Structure

Didactic: 15 months

Clinical: 12 months

Rotations:
7 mandatory, 1 elective, 5 weeks each

Unique Program Features

Early Clinical Exposure: The program offers early patient contact to students during the didactic year to begin to correlate classroom learning with patient care.

IDAHO

IDAHO STATE UNIVERSITY

Idaho State University
Email: pa@isu.edu

921 S. 8th Avenue
Stop 8253
Pocatello, ID 83209
Phone: 208-282-4726

Mission: The mission of the Idaho State University Physician Assistant program is to train PAs through service-oriented, multimodal, innovative learning. Graduates from ISUs PA Program will be highly competent, compassionate health care providers dedicated to serving individuals and their communities.

Accreditation:
Continued

Degree Offered:
Master (MPAS)

Start Date:
August annually

Program Length:
24 months

Class Capacity:
72 students

Tuition:
In-state: $20,352;
Out-of-state: $62,166;
Caldwell students: $55,200

GPA Requirement:
Prerequisite GPA: 3.0

Healthcare Experience:
Preferred, not required

PA Shadowing: Not required

Required Standardized Testing: GRE

Letters of Recommendation: Three required; no one specific

Seat Deposit: $750

CASPA Participant: Yes

Supplemental Application: Yes

Admissions: Not specified

Application Deadline:
November 1

Class of 2017
Male: 49%
Female: 51%
Minority: 16%
Prerequisite GPA: 3.82
GRE Verbal: 77th percentile
GRE Quantitative: 61st percentile
GRE Analytical: not reported
Faculty to Student Ratio: not reported
Average Healthcare Experience: not reported

PANCE Scores
5-year First Time Pass: 96%
Most Recent First Time Pass: 93%

Curriculum Structure
Didactic: 12 months
Clinical: 12 months
Rotations:
7 mandatory, 1 elective, duration not specified
Capstone Project: required for graduation

Prerequisite Coursework

Microbiology, Biochemistry, Human Anatomy, Human Psychology, Statistics, Abnormal Psychology or Developmental Psychology throughout the lifespan. Applicants maay have two courses in progress during spring of the year they enter the program, and all must be completed in the last 10 years.

Unique Program Features

Medical Spanish: Students can pursue individual Spanish for Healthcare Professions courses or complete a nine credit sequence to earn a graduate certificate in Spanish for Healthcare Professions.

International Activity: Students can participate in medical missions to the Dominican Republic or Peru and in an international rotation in Belize as part of their training.

One Program, Three Campuses: The program is offered simultaneously on three campuses in Pocatello, Meridian, and Caldwell to encompass the total 72 student class size.

ILLINOIS

MIDWESTERN UNIVERSITY (DOWNERS GROVE)

Midwestern University
Email:
admissil@midwestern.edu

555 31st Street
Downers Grove, IL 60515
Phone: 630-515-6034

Mission: The mission of the Midwestern University Physician Assistant (PA) Program is to develop competent and compassionate physician assistants who will make meaningful contributions to their patients, community, and profession.

Accreditation:
Continued

Degree Offered:
Master (MMS)

Start Date:
June annually

Program Length:
27 months

Class Capacity:
86 students

Tuition: $99,032

GPA Requirement:
Overall GPA 2.75;
Science GPA 2.75;

Healthcare Experience:
Preferred, not required

PA Shadowing:
Not required

Required Standardized Testing: GRE

Letters of Recommendation: Two required; no one specific

Seat Deposit: $750

CASPA Participant: Yes

Supplemental Application: No

Admissions: Rolling

Application Deadline:
October 1

Class of 2017
Male: 23%
Female: 77%
Minority:
not reported
GPA: 3.73
Science GPA: 3.70
GREVerbal: 66th percentile
GRE Quantitative:
63rd percentile
GRE Writing:
66th percentile
Faculty to Student Ratio: not reported
Average Healthcare Experience:
not reported

PANCE Scores
5-year First Time Pass:
99%
Most Recent First Time Pass: 100%

Curriculum Structure
Didactic: 12 months
Clinical: 12 months
Rotations:
8 mandatory,
2 electives;
4-6 weeks each
Capstone Project:
Required for graduation

Unique Program Features

Diverse Rotations: Students will be assigned to rotations that exemplify the geographic and demographic diversity of the region including inpatient and outpatient settings as well as rotations in urban, suburban, and rural communities.

Prerequisite Coursework

Biology with lab (4 credits), Anatomy (4 credits), General Chemistry with lab (4 credits), Organic Chemistry with lab (8 credits), Math (3 credits), Statistics (3 credits), English Composition (6 credits), Social and Behavioral Sciences (6 credits). All courses must be completed by Dec 31st of the year you apply.

Class of 2017

Male: 17%
Female: 83%
Minority: 10%
GPA: 3.73
Science GPA: 3.67
Prerequisite GPA: 3.84
GREVerbal: 79th percentile
GRE Quantitative: 72nd percentile
GRE Writing: 4.5
Faculty to Student Ratio: not reported
Average Healthcare Experience: 3,932 hours

PANCE Scores

5-year First Time Pass: 97% (based on four years of data)

Most Recent First Time Pass: 100%

Curriculum

Structure

Didactic: 12 months
Clinical: 12 months
Rotations: 7 mandatory, 4 electives; 4 weeks each
Capstone Project: Required for graduation

Northwestern University
Email: paprogram@northwestern.edu

240 E. Huron Street
Suite 1-200
Chicago, IL 60611
Phone: 312-503-1851

Mission: The mission of the Northwestern University Feinberg School of Medicine Physician Assistant (PA) Program is to prepare PAs to provide compassionate, high quality, patient-centered care as members of interdisciplinary teams. The graduates will be culturally competent, committed to continuous learning and professional development, and make significant contributions to communities and the advancement of the PA profession.

Accreditation: Continued
Degree Offered: Master (MMS)
Start Date: June annually
Program Length: 24 months
Class Capacity: 30 students
Tuition: $83,286

GPA Requirement: Overall GPA 2.8
Healthcare Experience: 1,000 hours recommended
PA Shadowing: Preferred, not required
Required Standardized Testing: GRE
Letters of Recommendation: Three required; no one specific
Seat Deposit: $1,000

CASPA Participant: Yes
Supplemental Application: Yes

Admissions: Rolling
Application Deadline: October 1

Unique Program Features

Problem Based Learning: This program utilizes problem based learning for much of the didactic curriculum. Students work in small groups of 6-8 students on a clinical problem and attempt to solve it, as well as identify their strengths and weaknesses in terms of clinical knowledge. Students also collaborate with medical students to solve simulated cases.

Student Profiles: These are available on the website to learn more about the program from a student perspective.

Facilities: The program is part of the Northwestern Medical Center in which students have 24 hours access to world-class facilities including an anatomy laboratory, simulation technology and immersive learning center, clinical education center, health-sciences library, small group rooms, and several of the area top hospitals for clinical learning.

Prerequisite Coursework

Biochemistry (3 credits), Microbiology (3 credits), Statistics (3 credits), Medical Terminology (1-3 credits), Anatomy and Physiology (6 credits). At most two prerequisites can be in progress during the fall prior to admission and one the spring prior to admission.

ROSALIND FRANKLIN UNIVERSITY OF MEDICINE

Rosalind Franklin University
Email: PA.Admissions
@rosalindfranklin.edu

3333 Green Bay Road
North Chicago, IL 60064
Phone: 847-578-8686

Mission: The mission of the Physician Assistant Program is to educate and prepare competent, compassionate, and ethical physician assistant leaders who, as integral members of the inter-professional healthcare team, will provide quality medical care.

Accreditation: Continued

Degree Offered: Master (MS)

Start Date: May annually

Program Length: 24 months

Class Capacity: 67 students

Tuition: $69,648

Seat Deposit: $500

GPA Requirement: Overall GPA 2.75; Science GPA 2.75; Prerequisite GPA 2.0

Healthcare Experience: Preferred, not required

PA Shadowing: Preferred, not required

Required Standardized Testing: GRE

Letters of Recommendation: Two required; one should be from an instructor who can attest to the applicant's scholastic aptitude, and one should be from a health care professional with whom the applicant has worked.

CASPA Participant: Yes

Supplemental Application: Yes

Admissions: Rolling

Application Deadline: December 1

Class of 2017

Male: not reported
Female: not reported
Minority: not reported
GPA: 3.45
Science GPA: 3.35
GREVerbal: not reported
GRE Quantitative: not reported
GRE Writing: not reported
Faculty to Student Ratio: not reported
Average Healthcare Experience: not reported

PANCE Scores
5-year First Time Pass: 96%
Most Recent First Time Pass: 95%

Curriculum Structure
Didactic: 12 months
Clinical: 12 months
Rotations: 6 mandatory, 2 electives; 6 weeks each
Master's Project: Required for graduation

Unique Program Features

Community Service: PA students participate in several activities in the community, such as Kid's First Health Fair, Healthy Families Clinic, Inter-professional Community Clinic, and Community Care Connection.

Research Day: Students deliver poster presentations of their Master's projects as part of the University-wide Research day each spring.

Prerequisite Coursework

Biochemistry (3 credits), Human Anatomy (3 credits), Human Physiology (3 credits), Introduction to Psychology (3 credits), Microbiology (3 credits). You may have up to three outstanding courses at the time of application.

Class of 2018

Male: 30%

Female: 70%

Minority: not reported

GPA: 3.58

Science GPA: 3.54

GRE Total: 308

Faculty to Student Ratio: not reported

Average Healthcare Experience: 2,204 hours

PANCE Scores

5-year First Time Pass: 100% (based on three years of data)

Most Recent First Time Pass: 100%

Curriculum Structure

Didactic: 12 months

Clinical: 21 months

Rotations: 8 mandatory, 1 electives, 3 advanced practice rotations; 4-10 weeks each

Master's Project: required for graduation

RUSH UNIVERSITY

RUSH UNIVERSITY
EMAIL:
PA_ADMISSIONS@RUSH.EDU

600 S. PAULINA STREET
SUITE 746 AAC
CHICAGO, IL 60612
PHONE: 312-563-3234

Mission: The mission of the physician assistant program is to train qualified, advanced practice physician assistants to practice medicine with competence, professionalism, and compassion driven by academic excellence in scholarship and research, and a spirit of service to the community.

Accreditation: Continued

Degree Offered: Master (MSPAS)

Start Date: June annually

Program Length: 33 months

Class Capacity: 30 students

Tuition: $94,950

GPA Requirement: Overall GPA 3.0; Science GPA 3.0;

Healthcare Experience: 1,000 hours required

PA Shadowing: Not required

Required Standardized Testing: GRE (302 minimum score)

Letters of Recommendation: Three required; no one specific

Seat Deposit: $250

CASPA Participant: Yes

Supplemental Application: Yes

Admissions: Rolling

Application Deadline: December 1

Prerequisite Coursework

Human Anatomy (3 credits), Human Physiology (3 credits), Biochemistry (3 credits), Microbiology (3 credits), Psychology (3 credits), Statistics (3 credits). It is strongly recommended that all courses be completed within seven years prior to application, and all science courses are required to be taken within 7 years prior to application. Candidates must have completed at least four prerequisites before applying.

Unique Program Features

Advanced Practice Rotations: Students complete 9 months of advanced clinical rotations where they choose a single, focused area of practice to hone their skills in and improve patient management prior to graduation.

Community Service: Each class of 30 students on average completes a total of 1025 hours of community service and medical mission work during their time at Rush.

SOUTHERN ILLINOIS UNIVERSITY

SIU PA Program

Email: paadvisement-L @listserv.siu.edu

600 Agriculture Drive

Carbondale, IL 62901

Phone: 618-453-8851

Mission: The mission of the Southern Illinois University School of Medicine Physician Assistant Program is to prepare healthcare professionals to provide primary health care, especially to underserved populations in rural and health professional shortage areas. We will enhance this healthcare by preparing graduates who are interdependent medical providers, dedicated to both community and profession. The academic setting will foster creative thinking and communication skills in our pursuit of excellence.

Accreditation:
Continued

Degree Offered:
Master (MSPA)

Start Date:
June annually

Program Length:
26 months

Class Capacity:
40 students

Tuition:
In-state: $48,561;
Out-of-state: $95,391

GPA Requirement:
Overall GPA 3.2;
Science GPA 3.2;

Healthcare Experience:
2,000 hours preferred

PA Shadowing:
Not required

Required Standardized Testing: GRE or MCAT

Letters of Recommendation: Three required; no one specific

Seat Deposit: $500

CASPA Participant: Yes

Supplemental Application: Yes

Admissions: Rolling

Application Deadline:
December 1

Prerequisite Coursework

Medical Terminology (or passage of proficiency exam), Chemistry with lab (2 semesters), Psychology, Human Physiology, Human Anatomy, Microbiology with lab, General Biology or Genetics or Cell and Molecular Biology, Statistics, English Composition, Basic Cardiac Life Support.

No student statistics reported

PANCE Scores

5-year First Time Pass: 99%

Most Recent First Time Pass: 100%

Curriculum Structure

Didactic: 12 months

Clinical: 14 months

Rotations:
8 mandatory,
1 elective,
1 preceptorship;
duration not specified

Master's Project:
required for graduation

Unique Program Features

Elective Coursework: The program offers both independent study and holistic medicine elective courses.

Problem Based Learning: The program utilizes problem based learning in didactic and clinical years. The PBL cases used are based on real patient problems that are carefully selected by faculty to stimulate students' learning in all relevant areas of basic clinical and behavioral sciences.

INDIANA

BUTLER UNIVERSITY

Butler University
College of Pharmacy
and Health Sciences

Email: PAadmissions@butler.edu

4600 Sunset Avenue

Indianapolis, IN 46208

Phone: 317-940-6529

Mission: To produce graduates with a foundation in primary care to deliver high quality, patient-centered care in a wide variety of clinical settings.

Accreditation:
Continued

Degree Offered:
Master (MPAS)

Start Date:
May annually

Program Length:
24 months

Class Capacity:
75 students

Tuition:
$80,000

GPA Requirement:
Overall GPA 3.4

Healthcare Experience:
Preferred, not required

PA Shadowing:
Not required

Required Standardized Testing: GRE

Letters of Recommendation: none required

Seat Deposit: $1,000

CASPA Participant: Yes

Supplemental Application: No

Admissions: Non-rolling

Application Deadline:
August 1

Prerequisite Coursework

General Chemistry with lab (2 semesters), Organic Chemistry with lab, Additional Chemistry course at 300 level or above, Biology at 200 level or above (5 semesters), Statistics or Biostatistics, Social Sciences (2 semesters).

No student statistics reported

PANCE Scores

5-year First Time Pass: 96%

Most Recent First Time Pass: 100%

Curriculum Structure

Didactic: 12 months
Clinical: 14 months
Rotations: 10 mandatory, 1 elective, 4 weeks each

Unique Program Features

Inter-professional Education Rotation: Students complete a week long clinical experience with a provider from a different specialty (nursing, physical therapy, etc) to learn from, with, and about another member of the healthcare team.

Military Seat: At least one seat in each PA class is reserved for a veteran or active military member.

Advocacy: Butler PA students and faculty have opportunities to lobby the Indiana General Assembly and U.S. Congress to promote expanded roles in healthcare for PAs

Class of 2017

Male: not reported

Female: not reported

Minority: not reported

GPA: 3.52

Science GPA: 3.46

GREVerbal: 151

GRE Quantitative: 153

GRE Writing: 4.0

Faculty to Student Ratio: not reported

Average Healthcare Experience: not reported

PANCE Scores

5-year First Time Pass: 90% (based on three years of data)

Most Recent First Time Pass: 97%

Curriculum Structure

Didactic: 15 months

Clinical: 12 months

Rotations: 9 mandatory, 2 elective, 4 weeks each

INDIANA STATE UNIVERSITY

Indiana State University
Email:
isu-amr@mail.indstate.edu

567 N. 5th Street
Terre Haute, IN 47809
Phone: not provided

Mission: The mission of the Indiana State University Physician Assistant Program is to create a student-centered educational environment that engages individuals to become compassionate, competent physician assistants who possess the clinical skills to contribute positively to the dynamic health care needs of rural and underserved populations.

Accreditation: Probation

Degree Offered: Master (MSPAS)

Start Date: January annually

Program Length: 27 months

Class Capacity: 30 students

Tuition: In-state: $36,084; Out-of-state: $70,866

GPA Requirement: Overall GPA 3.0; Prerequisite GPA 2.7

Healthcare Experience: Preferred, not required

PA Shadowing: Not required

Required Standardized Testing: GRE or MCAT

Letters of Recommendation: Three required; no one specific

Seat Deposit: $1,000

CASPA Participant: Yes

Supplemental Application: Yes

Admissions: Not specified

Application Deadline: March 1

Unique Program Features

Admissions Preference: Preference is given to residents of Indiana, Indiana State University graduates, and those interested in Rural Health Medicine (program has partnership with the Rural Health Innovation Collaborative

Inter-professional Education: PA students interact with physical therapy, nursing, athletic training and medical students throughout their education.

Prerequisite Coursework

Human Anatomy with lab, Human Physiology with lab, Microbiology with lab, Organic Chemistry I and II with lab, Statistics, Medical Terminology, Two Upper Level Biological Sciences courses. Courses must be completed by the summer before beginning the program

INDIANA UNIVERSITY SCHOOL OF HEALTH AND REHABILITATION SCIENCES

Indiana University School of Health and Rehabilitation Sciences

Email: Paadmit@iupui.edu

Coleman Hall, Room CF120
1140 W. Michigan Street
Indianapolis, IN 46202-5119
Phone: 317-278-9550

Mission: The mission of the Indiana University Master of Physician Assistant Studies program is to prepare students for physician assistant practice, with a focus on urban and rural underserved communities in the state of Indiana, using an inter-professional team approach to education.

Accreditation:
Provisional

Degree Offered:
Master (MPAS)

Start Date:
May annually

Program Length:
27 months

Class Capacity:
44 students

Tuition:
In-state: $57,511;
Out-of-state: $84,575

GPA Requirement:
Overall GPA 3.0;
Math/Science Prerequisite
GPA 3.2

Healthcare Experience:
500 hours required

PA Shadowing:
10 hours required

Required Standardized Testing: GRE

Letters of Recommendation: Two required; one from a PA

Seat Deposit: $500

CASPA Participant: Yes

Supplemental Application: Yes

Admissions: Rolling

Application Deadline:
September 1

PANCE Scores

5-year First Time Pass: N/A (only one year of data)

Most Recent First Time Pass: 90%

Curriculum Structure

Didactic: 15 months
Clinical: 12 months
Rotations:
9 mandatory,
2 elective, 1 medical subspecialty;
4 weeks each

Research Project: required for graduation

Unique Program Features

Admissions Preference: Indiana residents who live in medically underserved counties as well as military veterans are given preference points added to their total score during application review.

Prerequisite Coursework

Human Anatomy with lab, Human Physiology with lab, Microbiology with lab, General Chemistry with lab (2 semesters), Statistics or Biostatistics, General Biology I with lab, Other Human Biology with lab, Organic Chemistry with lab, Introductory Psychology, Medical Terminology.

University of Saint Francis
Email: dlabarbera@sf.edu

2701 Spring Street
Fort Wayne, IN 46808
Phone: 260-399-7700

Mission: The Department of Physician Assistant Studies provides education in medical knowledge and skills needed by individuals to serve effectively as mid-level practitioners with a special focus on meeting the needs of underserved populations. The Department prepares students to be clinicians who achieve professional standards and have enhanced critical thinking, clinical, and research skills. We offer an educational environment of mutual respect, personal growth, and professional advancement.

Accreditation: Continued

Degree Offered: Master (MSPAS)

Start Date: May annually

Program Length: 27 months

Class Capacity: 25 students

Tuition: $88,550

GPA Requirement: Overall GPA 3.0; Science GPA 2.85; Prerequisite GPA 2.0

Healthcare Experience: Required, no minimum amount

PA Shadowing: Not required

Required Standardized Testing: GRE

Letters of Recommendation: Two required; no one specific

Seat Deposit: $1,000

CASPA Participant: Yes

Supplemental Application: Yes

Admissions: Not specified

Application Deadline: December 1

Prerequisite Coursework

Chemistry (12 credits to include General, Organic, and Biochemistry), Biology (15 credits to include human anatomy, physiology, and microbiology), Psychology (6 credits)

No student statistics reported

PANCE Scores

5-year First Time Pass: 100%

Most Recent First Time Pass: 100%

Curriculum Structure

Didactic: 15 months

Clinical: 12 months

Rotations: 8 mandatory, 1 elective, 3 specialty track; 4 weeks each

Unique Program Features

Specialty Tracks: Students can choose a specialty track for their clinical rotations enabling them to complete a series of rotations in either trauma or surgery, hospital-based care, family practice, or internal medicine.

Student Profiles: The website lists profiles of each current student so prospective applicants can get a greater sense of what the admissions committee is looking for.

Problem Based Learning: The program uses problem based learning as the exclusive method of teaching for its medicine and therapeutics courses in the third and fourth semester of the program.

KANSAS

WICHITA STATE UNIVERSITY

Wichita State University
Email:
physician.assistant@wichita.edu

1845 Fairmount Street
Wichita, KS 67260
Phone: 316-978-3011

Mission: The mission of the Department of Physician Assistant is to be a learning community dedicated to developing generalist health care professionals by: Valuing students; Integrating teaching, scholarship, practice, and service; and partnering with the community.

Accreditation:
Continued

Degree Offered:
Master (MPA)

Start Date:
June annually

Program Length:
26 months

Class Capacity:
48 students

Tuition:
In-state: $25,792;
Out-of-state: $57,718

GPA Requirement:
Overall GPA 3.0;
Science GPA 3.0

Healthcare Experience:
Preferred, not required

PA Shadowing: Not required

Required Standardized Testing: none

Letters of Recommendation:
Three required; no one specific

Seat Deposit: $500

Class of 2017

Male: not reported
Female: not reported
Minority:
not reported
GPA: 3.60
Science GPA:
not reported
GRE: not required
Faculty to Student Ratio: not reported
Average Healthcare Experience:
not reported

PANCE Scores

5-year First Time Pass: 96%

Most Recent First Time Pass: 98%

Curriculum Structure

Didactic: 13 months
Clinical: 13 months
Rotations: 8 rotations, duration not specified

CASPA Participant: Yes

Supplemental Application: Yes

Admissions: Not specified

Application Deadline:
October 1

Prerequisite Coursework

Chemistry (12 credits), Biology to include Microbiology with lab (9 credits), Human Anatomy and Physiology with lab (5 credits), Statistics (3 credits), Psychology (3 credits), Medical Terminology (1 credit). All science prerequisites must be completed at time of application and all courses should be less than 10 years old.

Unique Program Features

Research Curriculum: The program has arguably the strongest record of student research and publication in the nation with over 40 publications from students working with faculty over the last 5 years.

Service Learning: Every student performs volunteer community service including Senior Mentor Program; Give-Kids-a-Smile fluoride varnish clinic; United Way Homeless Count; Ready Set Fit health education for elementary children; Sports Physicals provided for free at a socioeconomically disadvantaged rural county; and many others.

Primary Care and Rural/Underserved Focus: Every student gets to know their community by completing at least 12 weeks of rotations in primary care and 12 weeks in rural areas.

KENTUCKY

SULLIVAN UNIVERSITY

Sullivan University
Email:
PAProgram@sullivan.edu

2100 Gardiner Lane
Louisville, KY 40202
Phone: 502-413-8659

Mission: The Mission of Sullivan University Physician Assistant Program is to educate medical professionals who will be able to: Provide ethical, high quality and compassionate healthcare as part of an inter-professional team; Expand the concept of the Physician Assistant profession to the Commonwealth of Kentucky; Increase access to healthcare services to underserved populations

Demonstrate commitment to lifelong learning and participation in professional associations; Acknowledge and understand diversity in providing healthcare; and promote community involvement amongst faculty, staff and students.

Accreditation:
Provisional

Degree Offered:
Master (MSPA)

Start Date:
May annually

Program Length:
24 months

Class Capacity:
35 students

Tuition: $72,000

GPA Requirement:
Overall GPA 3.0;
Science GPA 3.0;
Prerequisite GPA 3.0

Healthcare Experience:
500 hours required

PA Shadowing:
Not required

Required Standardized Testing: None

Letters of Recommendation:
Three required; one from a physician or PA

Seat Deposit: $500

CASPA Participant: No

Supplemental Application: No

Admissions: Rolling

Application Deadline:
October 31

Prerequisite Coursework

Human Anatomy, Human Physiology, Microbiology, General Chemistry I and II with lab, Statistics, Introduction to Psychology or Developmental Psychology or Abnormal Psychology, English Composition or Communications, Medical Terminology. Up to two courses may be in progress at the time of application.

No class statistics reported

PANCE Scores

5-year First Time Pass:
N/A

Most Recent First Time Pass: N/A (have not graduated a class yet)

Curriculum Structure

Didactic: 12 months

Clinical: 12 months

Rotations:
7 mandatory,
1 elective; 6 weeks each.

Capstone Project:
Required for graduation

Unique Program Features

Curriculum Variety:
The curriculum uses a variety of teaching methodologies including asynchronous learning, case-based learning, early clinical exposure, problem based learning, and hybrid courses.

UNIVERSITY OF KENTUCKY

University of Kentucky
Email:
CHS-Admissions@uky.edu

900 South Limestone Street
Charles T. Wethington Building, Room 205
Lexington , KY 40536
Phone: 859-218-0492

Mission: To provide excellence in Physician Assistant education by training compassionate physician assistants who strive to provide the best medical care possible to people of the Commonwealth and beyond.

Accreditation: Continued

Degree Offered: Master (MSPAS)

Start Date: January annually

Program Length: 29 months

Class Capacity: 56 students

Tuition:
In-state: $43,932;
Out-of-state: $94,885

GPA Requirement: Overall GPA 2.75

Healthcare Experience: Required, no specific minimum

PA Shadowing: 50 hours required

Required Standardized Testing: GRE

Letters of Recommendation: Three required; one from a physician or PA, one from an academic advisor, and one from a physician or PA or an academic advisor.

Seat Deposit: $300

CASPA Participant: Yes

Supplemental Application: Yes

Admissions: Not specified

Application Deadline: July 15

Unique Program Features

Two Campuses: This program operates with 40 students at the Lexington Campus and 16 students at the Morehead State site. Students complete the same requirements for graduation and have dedicated faculty members at each location.

International Rotations: The program offers rotations in various countries including Kenya, Swaziland, and England, as well as opportunities to travel on shorter trips to Ecuador and Mexico.

Prerequisite Coursework

General Chemistry I and II with lab, Organic Chemistry w/lab, Human Anatomy and Physiology I and II with lab, General Biology with lab, Microbiology with lab, Statistics, Psychology, Developmental Psychology, Anthropology or Sociology, Medical Terminology (at least 2 credits). Two courses may be in progress at the time of application but must be completed by August 6, 2016.

UNIVERSITY OF THE CUMBERLANDS

University of the Cumberlands

Master of Science in Physician Assistant Studies Program

7985 College Station Drive
Williamsburg, KY 40769
Phone: 606-539-4616
Email: pa@ucumberlands.edu

PANCE Scores

5-year First Time Pass: N/A

Most Recent First Time Pass: N/A (have not graduated a class yet)

Mission: The mission of the Physician Assistant Program is to educate and prepare competent, compassionate, and committed Physician Assistant leaders who, as integral members of the modern professional healthcare team, are driven by academic excellence and will be servant leaders in their communities. The faculty and staff of the Physician Assistant Program will provide academic and clinical excellence in an environment of compassion and team cooperation, seeking to prepare clinicians for a lifelong commitment to continuing education, leadership, and medical service.

Curriculum Structure

Didactic: 15 months
Clinical: 12 months
Rotations: 9 mandatory, 1 elective rotation; 4-8 weeks each.
Capstone Project: Required for graduation

Unique Program Features

Not specified

Accreditation: Provisional

Degree Offered: Master (MSPAS)

Start Date: January annually

Program Length: 27 months

Class Capacity: 30 students

Tuition: $81,550

GPA Requirement: Overall GPA 3.0; Science GPA 3.0; Prerequisite GPA 3.0

Healthcare Experience: 500 hours required.

PA Shadowing: 50 hours required

Required Standardized Testing: GRE (score >300 is considered competitive)

Letters of Recommendation: Three required; two letters from medical providers and one academic letter

Seat Deposit: $500

CASPA Participant: Yes

Supplemental Application: Yes

Admissions: Not specified

Application Deadline: September 1

Prerequisite Coursework

Anatomy with lab (3 credits), Physiology with lab (3 credits), Microbiology with lab (3 credits), Medical Terminology, Upper Level Biology (6 credits), General Chemistry I and II with labs (6 credits), Organic Chemistry I or Biochemistry, Psychology (3 credits), Statistics (3 credits). The majority of coursework should be completed prior to application and all should be completed in the last 10 years.

LOUISIANA

LOUISIANA STATE UNIVERSITY – NEW ORLEANS

Louisiana State University
Health Science Center
Email:
PaProgram@lsuhsc.edu

411 South Prieur
LSUHSC-NO
New Orleans, LA 70112
Phone: 504-556-3420

Mission: : The Mission of the Louisiana State University Health Sciences Center- New Orleans Master of Physician Assistant Studies Program is to recruit and educate individuals of the highest quality from diverse backgrounds to provide evidence-based, patient-centered healthcare with compassion to the people of Louisiana.

Accreditation:
Provisional

Degree Offered:
Master (MPAS)

Start Date:
January annually

Program Length:
29 months

Class Capacity:
30 students

Tuition:
In-state: $51,813
(fees included);
Out-of-state: $106,154
(fees included)

GPA Requirement:
Overall GPA 3.0;
Science GPA 3.0

Healthcare Experience:
80 hours required

PA Shadowing:
Recommended, not required

Required Standardized Testing: GRE (minimum 153 quantitative, 144 verbal and 3.5 analytical)

Letters of Recommendation: Three required; one from a PA, two from an employer or course instructor

Seat Deposit: $500

CASPA Participant: Yes

Supplemental Application: No

Admissions: Not specified

Application Deadline:
August 1

Prerequisite Coursework

Biological Sciences I and II with lab (8 credits, Microbiology or Bacteriology with lab (3-4 credits), Chemistry I and II with labs (8 credits), Anatomy with lab (4 credits), Physiology with lab (3-4 credits), Statistics (3 credits), Genetics (3 credits), Organic Chemistry or Biochemistry (3-4 credits), Behavioral Sciences (6 credits), College Algebra or higher (3 credits), CPR. Courses must be completed in the last 10 years.

Class of 2017

Male: not reported
Female: not reported
Minority: not reported
GPA: 3.49
Science GPA: 3.47
GRE: not reported
Faculty to Student Ratio: not reported
Average Healthcare Experience: 2,600 hours

PANCE Scores

5-year First Time Pass: N/A (only one year of data)

Most Recent First Time Pass: 90%

Curriculum Structure

Didactic: 17 months

Clinical: 12 months

Rotations:
7 mandatory,
1 electives,
1 preceptorship;
4-8 weeks each

Master's Project:
required for graduation

Unique Program Features

Admissions Preference: The school has preference for applicants who are Louisiana residents.

No class statistics reported

PANCE Scores

5-year First Time Pass: not reported

Most Recent First Time Pass: 100%

Curriculum Structure

Didactic: 12 months

Clinical: 15 months

Rotations: 9 mandatory, 3 electives, 1 preceptorship; 4-8 weeks each

Master's Project: required for graduation

Unique Program Features

Admissions Preference: The school has preference for applicants who are Louisiana residents.

LSUHSC PA Program
Email: PAProgramShreveport@lsuhsc.edu

1501 Kings Highway
PO Box 33932
Shreveport, LA 71130
Phone: 318-813-2920

Mission: The mission of the PA Program is to provide a primary care curriculum to prepare competent Physician Assistant health care providers for Louisiana.

Accreditation: Continued

Degree Offered: Master (MPAS)

Start Date: May annually

Program Length: 27 months

Class Capacity: 38 students

Tuition: In-state $46,354 (fees included); Out-of-state: $72,287 (fees included)

GPA Requirement: Overall GPA 2.9

Healthcare Experience: 80 hours required

PA Shadowing: Recommended, not required

Required Standardized Testing: GRE (minimum 286)

Letters of Recommendation: Three required; no one specific

Seat Deposit: $150

CASPA Participant: Yes

Supplemental Application: Yes

Admissions: Not specified

Application Deadline: October 1

Prerequisite Coursework

Anatomy with lab (4 credits), Physiology (3 credits), Microbiology (4 credits), Chemistry with lab (8 credits), Upper Level Biology (8 credits), Statistics (3 credits), Medical Terminology (3 credits). Courses can be in progress at time of application.

OUR LADY OF THE LAKE COLLEGE

Our Lady of the Lake College
Email: not reported

5414 Brittany Drive
Baton Rouge, LA 70808
Phone: 225-768-1700

Mission: The purpose of the Physician Assistant (PA) program is to educate outstanding physician assistants who, together with physicians and allied health professionals, will provide quality healthcare to the residents of Louisiana and other states.

Accreditation:
Continued

Degree Offered:
Master (MMS)

Start Date:
January annually

Program Length:
28 months

Class Capacity:
30 students

Tuition:
$94,500 (approximate)

GPA Requirement: None

Healthcare Experience:
1,000 hours required

PA Shadowing:
Recommended shadowing three PAs, not required

Required Standardized Testing: GRE

Letters of Recommendation: Three required; one from a licensed PA, a previous employer, and a past College professor or advisor.

Seat Deposit: not reported

CASPA Participant: No

Supplemental Application: No

Admissions: Rolling

Application Deadline:
August 15

Prerequisite Coursework

Anatomy and Physiology I and II with lab, Microbiology, Organic Chemistry I, Organic Chemistry II or Biochemistry, Psychology, Statistics, Genetics. All must be completed by application deadline.

No class statistics reported

PANCE Scores

5-year First Time Pass: 83% (based on four years of data)

Most Recent First Time Pass: 81%

Curriculum Structure

Didactic: 16 months

Clinical: 12 months

Rotations:
9 mandatory, 1 elective, duration not specified

Master's Project: required for graduation

Unique Program Features

Application Process: Applicants must complete a short assessment of their knowledge of anatomy, physiology and biochemistry as part of the admissions process.

MAINE

UNIVERSITY OF NEW ENGLAND

University of New England
Email:
GradAdmissions@une.edu

716 Stevens Avenue
Portland, ME 04103
Phone: 207-221-4225

Mission: The mission of the University of New England Physician Assistant Program is to prepare masters level primary care Physician Assistants who will practice with physicians and other members of the health care team. The Program is committed to developing practitioners who are educated in all aspects of healthcare including geriatrics, health promotion and disease prevention, and public health practice. Special emphasis is placed on training clinicians who will provide primary healthcare to rural and urban underserved populations.

Accreditation:
Continuing

Degree Offered:
Master (MS)

Start Date:
May annually

Program Length:
24 months

Class Capacity:
50 students

Tuition: $40,620

CASPA Participant:
Yes

Supplemental Application: No

Admissions: Rolling

Application Deadline: October 1

GPA Requirement:
Overall GPA 3.0;
Science GPA 3.0

Healthcare Experience:
250 hours required

PA Shadowing: Required (no specific number of hours)—Applicants will be required to show evidence of PA shadowing hours in a primary care, inpatient or outpatient setting and must record in the "Health Care Shadowing Experience" section of CASPA.

Required Standardized Testing: GRE

Letters of Recommendation: Three required; not from anyone specific

Seat Deposit: $2,000

Class Statistics
GPA: 3.55
Science GPA: 3.50
Average Healthcare Experience:
2500-3500 hours

PANCE Scores
5-year First Time Pass: 96%

Most Recent First Time Pass: 98%

Curriculum Structure
Didactic: 12 months
Clinical: 12 months
Rotations:
6 mandatory,
1 primary care elective, 1 other elective (all 6 weeks)
Capstone Project: Not required

Unique Program Features

Community Service: Students have the opportunity to participate in many community service activities, including a mobile health van and mission trips to Ghana.

Direct Entry: They offer a pre-PA accelerated 3+2 track to earn a BS and MS in 5 years total.

Prerequisite Coursework

Biology with lab (2 semesters), General Chemistry with lab (2 semesters), Human Anatomy and Physiology with lab (2 semesters), Psychology or Sociology (2 semesters), English (2 semesters)

Prerequisites may be in-progress or planned at the time of application, but must be completed by December 31st, of the application year.

MARYLAND

ANNE ARUNDEL COMMUNITY COLLEGE

Anne Arundel Community College
Email:
healthprofessions@aacc.edu

Florestano 111
101 College Parkway
Arnold, MD 21012
Phone: 410-777-7310

Mission: To promote excellence in education in order to produce competent, ethical and compassionate health care providers who are ready to fulfill the roles and duties of the primary care physician assistant, recognize and promote the value of diversity, and who are committed to lifelong learning.

Accreditation:
Continuing

Degree Offered:
Certificate, Master (MSHS)

Start Date:
May annually

Program Length:
25 months

Class Capacity:
40 students

Tuition:
In-county: $37,340;
Out-of-county: $45,424;
Out-of-state: $71,501

GPA Requirement:
Overall GPA 3.0;
Science GPA 3.0;
Prerequisite GPA 3.0

Healthcare Experience:
1,400 hours required

PA Shadowing:
Not required

Required Standardized Testing: GRE

Letters of Recommendation: Three required; no one specific

Seat Deposit: $500

CASPA Participant: Yes

Supplemental Application: No

Admissions: Not specified

Application Deadline:
September 1

Class of 2017
Male: 28%
Female: 72%
Minority:
not reported
GPA: 3.53
Science GPA: 3.47
GRE Total:
not reported
Faculty to Student Ratio: not reported
Average Healthcare Experience:
4,284 hours

PANCE Scores

5-year First Time Pass:
98%

Most Recent First Time Pass: 100%

Curriculum Structure

Didactic: 12 months

Clinical: 13 months

Rotations: 9 total, other details not provided

Prerequisite Coursework

General Microbiology with lab (4 credits), Anatomy and Physiology I and II with lab (8 credits), General Chemistry I or General Chemistry II or Organic Chemistry or Biochemistry with lab (4 credits), Introduction to Psychology or Developmental Psychology or Human Growth and Development (3 credits), Elementary Statistics or Statistics in Social and Behavioral Sciences or Biostatistics (3 credits). All courses must be completed with a "B" or better. Anatomy and Physiology must have been taken in the last 7 years of the data the CASPA application is submitted.

Unique Program Features

University of Maryland: AACC has a partnership with the University of Maryland allowing students to take courses from both colleges to obtain the PA certificate and Master's degree in 25 months.

Primary Care Focus: The coursework is based in primary care and approximately 40% of graduates enter into the field.

No class statistics provided

PANCE Scores

5-year First Time Pass: 98%

Most Recent First Time Pass: 100%

Curriculum Structure

Didactic: 12 months

Clinical: 14 months

Rotations: 9 mandatory, 1 elective, unspecified duration

Unique Program Features

Towson University: The CCBC program collaborates with Towson University so that students can be awarded a Certificate as a PA and Master's degree (from Towson) upon graduation. Students take 36 graduate level credits from Towson during the program.

TOWSON UNIVERSITY /COMMUNITY COLLEGE OF BALTIMORE COUNTY

Towson University CCBC - Essex
Email: sshaw@ccbcmd.edu

7201 Rossville Boulevard
Administration Building - Room 101
Baltimore, MD 21237
Phone: 443-840-2854

Mission: The Towson University - CCBC Essex Physician Assistant Program provides a generalist foundation with a broad range of knowledge and skills to prepare competent PAs for practice in diverse medical settings.

Accreditation: Continuing

Degree Offered: Certificate, Master (MSPAS)

Start Date: June annually

Program Length: 26 months

Class Capacity: 36 students

Tuition: In-state: $24,000; Out-of-state: $51,000

GPA Requirement: Overall GPA 3.0; Prerequisite GPA 3.0

Healthcare Experience: 800 hours required (1,400 preferred)

PA Shadowing: Not required

Required Standardized Testing: None

Letters of Recommendation: Three required; one from a PA, physician, or professor

Seat Deposit: $2,600

CASPA Participant: Yes

Supplemental Application: Yes

Admissions: Rolling

Application Deadline: September 1

Prerequisite Coursework

Human Anatomy and Physiology (8 credits), Microbiology (4 credits), Essentials of Organic and Biochemistry (4 credits), Statistics (3 credits), Medical Terminology (3 credits). All must be completed with a "B" or better.

MASSACHUSETTS

BOSTON UNIVERSITY

Boston University
Email:
paoffice@bu.edu

72 East Concord Street
L 801
Boston, MA 2118
Phone: 617-638-5744

Mission: The mission of the Boston University School of Medicine Physician Assistant Program is to educate physician assistants who will produce exceptional outcomes while caring for a diverse population of patients, including those from vulnerable communities and to cultivate leaders who will advance the physician assistant profession. We value excellence, integrity, social justice, service, and are committed to developing a successful model for interprofessional education and clinical practice.

Accreditation:
Provisional

Degree Offered:
Master (MMSc)

Start Date:
April annually

Program Length:
28 months

Class Capacity:
36 students

Tuition: $94,898

CASPA Participant: Yes

Supplemental Application: Yes

Admissions: Not rolling

Application Deadline:
October 1

GPA Requirement:
No minimum overall GPA; 3.0 cumulative science GPA

Healthcare Experience:
Not required

PA Shadowing:
Not required

Required Standardized Testing: GRE required (scores must be above the 50th percentile)

Letters of Recommendation: Three required; One from a PA or MD, one from a former professor, and one from a former employer

Seat Deposit: $550

Class of 2016
Male: 43%
Female: 57%
Minority:
Not reported
GPA: 3.5
Science GPA: 3.4
GRE: Verbal – 59%; Quantitative – 69%; Writing – 67%
Faculty to Student Ratio: Not reported
Average Healthcare Experience:
Not reported

PANCE Scores
5-year First Time Pass: Not available yet

Most Recent First Time Pass: Not available yet

Curriculum Structure
Didactic: 12 months
Clinical: 16 months
Rotations:
7 mandatory (4-8 weeks long), 4 electives (4-5 weeks long)
Thesis: Required for graduation; 2 months during clinical year are dedicated to thesis work

Prerequisite Coursework

General Biology or Zoology with lab (1 semester), Human or Animal Physiology (1 semester), General Chemistry with lab (1 semester), Organic Chemistry with lab (1 semester), Biochemistry (1 semester)

3 upper level Biology courses (1 semester each). Online courses do not count towards prerequisite course requirements. Prerequisites may be in progress at the time of e-submission to CASPA but must be completed by the October 1 deadline.

Unique Program Features

Education: Novel interprofessional education approach with Medicine and Dentistry where students from each program complete a large portion of didactics together.

Rotations: International rotations available

Class Statistics
GPA: 3.3 – 3.5

PANCE Scores
5-year First Time Pass: 94%

Most Recent First Time Pass: 99%

Unique Program Features

Summer Break: The didactic part of the curriculum spans two years, with the summer following year 1 off.

Facilities: State-of-the-art patient assessment laboratory featuring the latest equipment and simulators is available for students to learn physical exam skills.

MCPHS University
Email: janis.chandler@mcphs.edu

179 Longwood Avenue
Boston, MA 02115
Phone: 617-274-3376

Mission: The mission of the MCPHS University Boston PA Program is to provide each student with the knowledge and skills to provide quality and compassionate medical care, function as a highly valued member of a health care team and serve as a patient advocate.

Accreditation: Continuing

Degree Offered: Master (MPAS)

Start Date: September annually

Program Length: 36 months

Class Capacity: 100 students

Tuition: $118,850

GPA Requirement: Overall GPA 3.0; Prerequisite GPA 3.0

Healthcare Experience: Preferred/Recommended (250-500 hours)

PA Shadowing: Not required

Required Standardized Testing: None

Letters of Recommendation: Three required; not from anyone specific

Seat Deposit: $500

CASPA Participant: Yes

Supplemental Application: No

Admissions: Rolling

Application Deadline: November 1

Prerequisite Coursework

General Biology I and II with lab (2 semesters), Human Physiology I and II (2 semesters), Microbiology with lab (1 semester), General Chemistry I and II with lab (2 semesters), Biochemistry (1 semester), Psychology (1 semester)

Statistics (1 semester). Math and science courses must be completed no more than ten years prior to the anticipated date of matriculation. Applicants cannot have more than 2 outstanding pre-requisites at the time of application.

MCPHS—WORCESTER AND MANCHESTER

MCPHS University—Worcester
19 Foster Street
Worcester, MA 01608
Phone: 508-373-5607
Email: admissions.worcester@mcphs.edu

MCPHS University—Manchester
1260 Elm Street
Manchester, NH 03101
Phone: 603-314-1701
Email: admissions.manchester@mcphs.edu

Mission: The program prepares highly qualified physician assistants who regardless of practice settings, are sensitive to both individual and cultural differences in the communities they serve. Through an integrated curriculum in the medical sciences and the healing arts, the program provides a comprehensive educational program that meets the demands of a dynamic healthcare system. As a community of learners, the program fosters professional growth through scholarly pursuit and practical experiences while promoting the integration of the whole person in the development of clinical, interpersonal, and professional skills required in the collaborative practice of medicine as physician assistants.

Accreditation: Continuing

Degree Offered: Master (MPAS)

Start Date: January annually

Program Length: 24 months

Class Capacity: 70 students

Tuition: $87,804

GPA Requirement: Overall GPA 2.75

Healthcare Experience: Preferred/Recommended (250-500 hours)

PA Shadowing: Recommended

Required Standardized Testing: None

Letters of Recommendation: Two required; not from anyone specific

Seat Deposit: $500

CASPA Participant: Yes

Supplemental Application: No

Admissions: Not reported

Application Deadline: March 1

No class statistics reported

PANCE Scores

5-year First Time Pass: 93%

Most Recent First Time Pass: 95%

Curriculum Structure

Didactic: 12 months

Clinical: 12 months

Rotations: 8 mandatory, 1 elective (all 5 weeks long)

Capstone Project: Required for graduation

Unique Program Features

Two Campuses: Lectures are provided on both campuses through state-of-the-art simultaneous video distance education.

Clinical Rotations: International rotations available.

Prerequisite Coursework

Human Anatomy and Physiology I and II with lab (2 semesters), Microbiology with lab (1 semester), General Chemistry I and II with lab (2 semesters), Organic Chemistry with lab (1 semester), Biochemistry (1 semester), Psychology (1 semester), Statistics (1 semester). Math and science courses must be completed no more than ten years prior to the anticipated date of matriculation.

PANCE Scores

None available yet

Curriculum Structure

Didactic: 12 months

Clinical: 13 months

Rotations: 7 mandatory, 2 elective (all 5 weeks long)

Capstone Project: Not required

Unique Program Features

Program Focus: Dedicated to primary care for urban, underserved populations

Facilities: On-site simulation and health assessment labs

MGH INSTITUTE OF HEALTH PROFESSIONS

MGH Institute of Health Professions
Email: pa@mghihp.edu

36 1st Avenue
Charlestown Navy Yard
Boston, MA 02129
Phone: 617-724-1839

Mission: The mission of the Master of Physician Assistant Studies Program (MPAS) at MGH Institute of Health Professions is to prepare compassionate and highly competent physician assistants to provide leadership in serving diverse communities and the profession, foster a commitment to excellence and advocacy, and contribute to evidence-based, interprofessional practice.

Accreditation: Provisional

Degree Offered: Master (MPAS)

Start Date: May annually

Program Length: 25 months

Class Capacity: 40 students

Tuition: $90,000

GPA Requirement: No minimums

Healthcare Experience: Required (1000 hours)—paid experience with hands-on patient care

PA Shadowing: Not reported

Required Standardized Testing: GRE or MCAT

Letters of Recommendation: Three required; not from anyone specific

Seat Deposit: $500

CASPA Participant: Yes

Supplemental Application: Yes

Admissions: Not reported

Application Deadline: August 1

Prerequisite Coursework

Human Anatomy and Physiology with lab (2 semesters) Biology with lab (1 semester) Chemistry with lab (1 semester) Chemistry with lab (2 semesters) Psychology (1 semester) Statistics (1 semester)

**Note: All prerequisites must be completed with a grade of "C" or better. There may be no more than 2 outstanding prerequisites at the time of application.

NORTHEASTERN UNIVERSITY

Northeastern University
Email:
paprogram@neu.edu

202 Robinson Hall
Boston, MA 02115
Phone: 617-373-3195

Mission: : The mission of the Northeastern University Physician Assistant Program is to prepare students to become exceptional clinicians and leaders within the health care community.

Accreditation:
Continuing

Degree Offered:
Master (MSPAS)

Start Date:
August annually

Program Length:
24 months

Class Capacity:
40 students

Tuition: $78,990

GPA Requirement: Overall GPA 3.0; Science GPA 3.0;

Healthcare Experience:
2,000 hours required

PA Shadowing:
Not required, but highly recommended

Required Standardized Testing: None

Letters of Recommendation: Three required; two should be from individuals that the applicant worked with while obtaining health care experience.

Seat Deposit: $500

CASPA Participant: Yes

Supplemental Application: Yes

Admissions: Not rolling

Application Deadline:
September 1

Prerequisite Coursework

Anatomy and Physiology (2 semesters), Biology (2 semesters) with lab (1 semester), Chemistry (2 semesters) with lab (1 semester), Statistics (1 semester).A grade of "B" or better is required for each prerequisite course.

PANCE Scores

5-year First Time Pass: 100%

Most Recent First Time Pass: 100%

Curriculum Structure

Didactic: 12 months

Clinical: 15 months

Rotations: 7 mandatory, 1 elective (each 6 weeks); 3 PA seminars during clinical year as well

Unique Program Features

Program Entry: There are two different entry points to the program, as a freshman college student (6 year program) or as a graduate student (2 year program).

Facilities: State-of-the-art medical simulation lab on-site.

Rotations: A six-week international medical Spanish elective rotation in Costa Rica is now available.

SPRINGFIELD COLLEGE

Springfield College
Email: lsaloio @springfieldcollege.edu

263 Alden Street
Springfield, MA 01109-3797
Phone: 413-748-3554

Mission: The mission of the Springfield College Physician Assistant Program is to educate students in spirit, mind, and body for leadership in clinical, community, and academic service to humanity by building upon its foundations of Humanities and academic excellence.

Accreditation: Continuing

Degree Offered: Master (MSPAS)

Start Date: January annually

Program Length: 27 months

Class Capacity: 35 students

Tuition: $106, 362

GPA Requirement: Overall GPA 3.0; Science GPA 3.0; Prerequisite GPA 3.0

Healthcare Experience: 470 hours required

PA Shadowing: Required (30 hours)—Cannot be a first-degree relative

Required Standardized Testing: Not required

Letters of Recommendation: Three required; One from an employer, one from a science professor, and one from a health care provider

Seat Deposit: $250

CASPA Participant: No

Supplemental Application: Yes

Admissions: Not reported

Application Deadline: June 1 (preferred April 1)

Prerequisite Coursework

Biology with lab, Human Anatomy and Physiology with lab, Microbiology, Organic Chemistry , General Chemistry with lab, Biochemistry, Statistics, Pre-Calculus (or other higher level math). Prerequisite courses must be completed by the end of the summer term prior to enrollment, with no more than two outstanding at the time of application.

TUFTS UNIVERSITY

Tufts University
Email:
paprogram@tufts.edu

136 Harrison Avenue
Suite 207
Boston, MA 02111
Phone: 617-636-0405

Mission: Our mission is to promote human health by providing excellent education to future physician assistants so that they are prepared to become integral members of the health care team. We fulfill this mission in a dynamic learning environment that emphasizes rigorous fundamentals, innovative delivery of the curriculum, and compassionate care to diverse patient populations. Our graduates will be prepared to participate in all aspects of the health care continuum, including disease management, health promotion and maintenance, and palliative care.

Accreditation:
Provisional

Degree Offered:
Master (MMS)

Start Date:
January annually

Program Length:
25 months

Class Capacity:
50 students

Tuition: $79,464

CASPA Participant: Yes

Supplemental Application: Yes

Admissions: Rolling

Application Deadline:
Recommended submission by July 1 for CASPA verification by August 1

GPA Requirement:
Overall GPA 3.2

Healthcare Experience:
1,000 hours required

PA Shadowing:
Encouraged, but not required and cannot be counted as direct patient care

Required Standardized Testing: GRE or MCAT

Letters of Recommendation:
Three required; at least one reference should be from a supervisor of a direct patient care experience and should substantiate the applicant's experience and performance

Seat Deposit: $1,000

Class of 2017
Male: 24%
Female: 76%
Minority: not reported
GPA: 3.57
Science GPA: 3.58
GRE: Verbal – 69%; Quantitative – 62%
Faculty to Student Ratio: not reported
Average Healthcare Experience: not reported

PANCE Scores
5-year First Time Pass: 100% (one class graduated so far)

Most Recent First Time Pass: 100%

Curriculum Structure
Didactic: 12 months
Clinical: 13 months
Rotations:
9 mandatory (4-8 weeks long), 2 elective (4 weeks long)
Capstone Project:
Required for graduation

Prerequisite Coursework

Human Anatomy and Physiology (2 semesters), Biology with lab (2 semesters)

Chemistry with lab (2 semesters; General and Organic accepted), Microbiology with lab (1 semester), Statistics (1 semester). All prerequisites must be completed at the time of application e-submission to CASPA.

Unique Program Features

Dual Degree: The program offers a 3 year combined PA/MPH option to students.

Community Service: The Sharewood Project is a free health care organization serving the medically underserved populations of the greater Boston area. Physician Assistant students have the opportunity to volunteer in the clinic alongside medical students and physicians. It is an opportunity to build clinical and interpersonal skills while giving back to this diverse patient population.

Facilities: Clinical Skills and Simulation Center – A state-of-the-art facility where students can gain hands on experience with new procedures before attempting them on a real patient. The 9,000-square-foot facility features three simulation rooms equipped with computerized mannequins. These mannequins are designed to model real patients as closely as possible and display symptoms and distress the same way humans do including sweating, changes in heart rate, coughing, etc.

MICHIGAN

CENTRAL MICHIGAN UNIVERSITY

Central Michigan University
Email: chpadmit@cmich.edu

1280 E. Campus Drive
HPB 1212
Mount Pleasant, MI 48859
Phone: 989-774-1730

Mission: The mission of the Central Michigan University Physician Assistant Program is to produce well-educated and highly-trained Physician Assistants who provide evidence-based medical services within the interdisciplinary primary care environment, with an emphasis on diversity and service to medically underserved populations in rural or urban communities.

Accreditation:
Probation

Degree Offered:
Master (MPAS)

Start Date:
May annually

Program Length:
27 months

Class Capacity:
34 students

Tuition:
In-state: $69,870;
Out-of-state: $100,940

GPA Requirement:
Overall GPA 3.25;
Prerequisite GPA 3.0

Healthcare Experience:
500 hours required

PA Shadowing:
Not required

Required Standardized Testing: GRE

Letters of Recommendation: Three required; no one specific

Seat Deposit: $1,000

CASPA Participant: Yes

Supplemental Application: Yes

Admissions: Not specified

Application Deadline:
September 1

Prerequisite Coursework

Anatomy with lab, Physiology with lab, Pathophysiology, Microbiology with or without lab, General Chemistry with lab, Organic Chemistry, Biochemistry, Introductory Psychology, Developmental Psychology, Statistics. Two courses can be in progress at the time of application and all courses must be completed by 12/31 of the application year. Courses must be less than six years old.

No class statistics reported

PANCE Scores
5-year First Time Pass: 96%

Most Recent First Time Pass: 95%

Curriculum Structure
Didactic: 15 months
Clinical: 12 months
Rotations:
7 mandatory,
1 electives;
5 weeks each

Unique Program Features

Early Clinical Exposure: In their first year, students spend one day per week seeing patients with a primary care preceptor for approximately 9 months. This allows them to hone their clinical skills and apply didactic information to patients as it is learned.

Fundamental Critical Care Support: The students complete the FCCS curriculum at the end of didactic year which provides them with procedural skills but also gives them the chance to take a specialty exam for certification in critical care medicine.

Class of 2017

Male: 20%

Female: 80%

Minority: not reported

GPA: 3.7

Science GPA: not reported

GRE: not required

Faculty to Student Ratio: not reported

Average Healthcare Experience: not reported

PANCE Scores

5-year First Time Pass: N/A

Most Recent First Time Pass: N/A (have not graduated first class yet)

Curriculum Structure

Didactic: 12 months

Clinical: 12 months

Rotations: 7 mandatory, 2 electives, 1 preceptorship; 4 weeks each (preceptorship 6 weeks)

EASTERN MICHIGAN UNIVERSITY

Eastern Michigan University
Email: chhs_paprogram@emich.edu

222 Rackham Building
Ypsilanti, MI 48197
Phone: 734-487-2843

Mission: The Eastern Michigan University Physician Assistant Program mission is to identify, train and support a diverse population of graduate students to become highly respected ambassadors of the profession and extraordinary healthcare providers with a strong foundation in primary care medicine and interdisciplinary practice.

Accreditation: Provisional

Degree Offered: Master (MSPAS)

Start Date: May annually

Program Length: 24 months

Class Capacity: 40 students

Tuition: In-state: $66,896; Out-of-state: $117,679 (fees included)

GPA Requirement: Overall GPA 3.0

Healthcare Experience: 500 hours required

PA Shadowing: Not required

Required Standardized Testing: None

Letters of Recommendation: Two required; no one specific

Seat Deposit: $1,000

CASPA Participant: Yes

Supplemental Application: Yes

Admissions: Not specified

Application Deadline: September 1

Unique Program Features

Multiple Teaching Styles: The program utilizes traditional lectures, problem-based learning, practical training, out of classroom learning and high fidelity medical simulation.

Facilities: There are newly renovated facilities for PA students including a human anatomy lab and advanced medical simulation center, as well as clinical skills laboratories, small group rooms, physical exam laboratory, advanced patient exam suites, a computer room, and a student lounge.

Prerequisite Coursework

Anatomy, Physiology, General Chemistry with lab, Organic Chemistry with lab or Biochemistry with lab, Microbiology with lab, Lifespan Psychology, Statistics. All courses must be at least 3 credits and completed with a "B-"or better in the last 10 years. Five out of seven must be completed at the time of the application and the other two must be completed by Jan 1st of the year you plan to start the program.

GRAND VALLEY STATE UNIVERSITY

Grand Valley State University
Email: pas@gvsu.edu

301 Michigan Street
Suite 113
Grand Rapids, MI 49503
Phone: 616-331-5700

Mission: The mission of the program is to educate individuals to become competent Physician Assistants, who possess the skills necessary for inter-professional medical practice

Accreditation: Continued

Degree Offered: Master (MPAS)

Start Date: August annually

Program Length: 28 months

Class Capacity: 48 students

Tuition:
In-state: $65,302;
Out-of-state: $84,872

GPA Requirement:
Overall GPA 3.0;
Science GPA 3.0;
Prerequisite GPA 3.0

Healthcare Experience: 500 hours required

PA Shadowing: Not required

Required Standardized Testing: GRE

Letters of Recommendation: Two required; one is recommended to be from a PA

Seat Deposit: None

CASPA Participant: Yes

Supplemental Application: No

Admissions: Not specified

Application Deadline: September 15

Prerequisite Coursework

General Biology, General Chemistry, Genetics, Organic Chemistry, Biochemistry, Human Anatomy, Human Physiology, Statistics, Psychology, Microbiology, Physics. Biochemistry, Human Anatomy, Human Physiology, and Microbiology must be taken less than 5 years ago. Anatomy, Physiology, Organic Chemistry, Biochemistry, and Microbiology must be completed at the time of application.

Unique Program Features

One Program, Two Locations: The program accepts up to 36 students on its Grand Rapids campus and 12 students on its Traverse City campus. The Traverse City students interact with the Grand Rapids lecturers and students through video conferencing.

Academic Medical Center: The main campus is located in the center of growing health complex which includes a med school, pharmacy school, 1000 bed hospital system with level 1 trauma center, cancer center, heart center, world class children's hospital and an international research institute.

International Rotation: Opportunities are available and can be counted as an elective.

Class of 2017

Male: not reported

Female: not reported

Minority: not reported

GPA: 3.62

Science GPA: not reported

GRE: 308 (verbal + quantitative)

Faculty to Student Ratio: not reported

Average Healthcare Experience: not reported

PANCE Scores

5-year First Time Pass: 98%

Most Recent First Time Pass: 100%

Curriculum Structure

Didactic: 16 months

Clinical: 12 months

Rotations: 8 mandatory, 1 elective, 1 preceptorship; 5 weeks each (elective 2 weeks, preceptorship 8 weeks)

UNIVERSITY OF DETROIT/MERCY

University of Detroit Mercy
Email: chpgrad@udmercy.edu

4001 West McNichols Road
CHP 115
Detroit, MI 48221-3038
Phone: 313-993-2474

Mission: The University of Detroit Mercy Physician Assistant Program is dedicated to the education of clinically competent medical professionals thoroughly prepared to deliver quality patient care in the context of a dynamic health care delivery system.

Accreditation: Continued

Degree Offered: Master (MS)

Start Date: August annually

Program Length: 24-36 months

Class Capacity: 40 students

Tuition: $93,337

GPA Requirement: Overall GPA 3.0; Science GPA 3.0; Prerequisite GPA 3.0

Healthcare Experience: 1,000 hours required

PA Shadowing: Not required

Required Standardized Testing: GRE (minimum combined score of 291)

Letters of Recommendation: Two required; one is recommended to be from a PA or physician

Seat Deposit: $1,000

CASPA Participant: Yes

Supplemental Application: Yes

Admissions: Not specified

Application Deadline: January 15

Unique Program Features

Part-Time Program: Students who wish to continue working during their training can enter the part-time track which is completed over 36 months. The didactic curriculum is divided into 2 years. Students then complete their rotations afterwards.

Admissions Preference: UDM undergraduates, applicants from under-served communities and underrepresented minorities in the profession may be given additional consideration in the application process.

Prerequisite Coursework

Nutrition, Medical Ethics, Statistics, Advanced Physiology, Microbiology, Developmental Psychology. Courses must have been completed in the past 6 years and all must be completed by the deadline of January 15.

WAYNE STATE UNIVERSITY

Wayne State University
Email: paadmit@wayne.edu

259 Mack Avenue
Suite 2590
Detroit, MI 48201
Phone: 313-577-1368

Mission: The mission of the Wayne State University Physician Assistant Studies program is to develop highly competent and passionate physician assistants who are deeply committed to the practice of medicine in a range of urban and underserved health care settings. The program exemplifies excellence and innovation in health care delivery and service to the community.

Accreditation:
Continued

Degree Offered:
Master (MSPAS)

Start Date:
May annually

Program Length:
24 months

Class Capacity:
50 students

Tuition:
In-state: $39,700;
Out-of-state: $74,949

CASPA Participant: Yes

Supplemental Application: Yes

Admissions: Not specified

Application Deadline:
September 1

GPA Requirement:
Overall GPA 3.0;
Prerequisite GPA 3.0

Healthcare Experience:
500 hours required

PA Shadowing:
Not required

Required Standardized Testing: GRE (minimum combined score of 285 and 3.5 on writing)

Letters of Recommendation: Three required; one of the three recommendations must be completed by an individual who has observed the applicant during direct patient contact experience

Seat Deposit: $500

Class of 2017
Male: 24%
Female: 76%
Minority: not reported
GPA: 3.75
Prerequisite GPA: 3.84
GRE Verbal: 153
GRE Quantitative: 152
GRE Writing: 4.2
Faculty to Student Ratio: not reported
Average Healthcare Experience: not reported

PANCE Scores
5-year First Time Pass: 96%

Most Recent First Time Pass: 98%

Curriculum Structure
Didactic: 12 months
Clinical: 12 months
Rotations:
7 mandatory,
1 preceptorship;
variable duration

Prerequisite Coursework

Human Anatomy, Human Physiology (2 courses), Microbiology with lab, Chemistry (2 courses, one must be Organic Chemistry or Biochemistry), Nutrition, Developmental Psychology, Basic Statistics, English Composition (2 courses), Medical Terminology. All courses must be completed by 9/1 of the year you apply.

Unique Program Features

Community Service: The program has an extensive history of community service working with medically underserved populations, Detroit public schools, Special Olympics Detroit, WSU Health Education for Longevity and Prevention Clinic, and other organizations selected by current students.

Class of 2017

Male: not reported

Female: not reported

Minority: not reported

GPA: 3.61

Prerequisite GPA: 3.60

GRE: not required

Faculty to Student Ratio: not reported

Average Healthcare Experience: 4,285

PANCE Scores

5-year First Time Pass: 93%

Most Recent First Time Pass: 95%

Curriculum Structure

Didactic: 12 months

Clinical: 12 months

Rotations: 7 mandatory, 0 electives; 4-8 weeks each

Master's Paper and Presentation: required for graduation

WESTERN MICHIGAN UNIVERSITY

Western Michigan University
Email: Not provided

1901 W. Michigan
Kalamazoo, MI 49007
Phone: 269-387-5311

Mission: The WMU Department of Physician Assistant is dedicated to educating competent, caring physician assistants to practice primary care medicine with the supervision of a physician, and to providing physician assistants to serve in all areas of society.

Accreditation: Continued

Degree Offered: Master (MS)

Start Date: September annually

Program Length: 24 months

Class Capacity: 40 students

Tuition:
In-state: $50,379;
Out-of-state: $106,708

GPA Requirement: Last 60 Credit Hour GPA: 3.0

Healthcare Experience: 1,000 hours required

PA Shadowing: Not required

Required Standardized Testing: None

Letters of Recommendation: Three required; no one specific

Seat Deposit: $750

CASPA Participant: Yes

Supplemental Application: Yes

Admissions: Not specified

Application Deadline: December 1

Unique Program Features

Community Service: The students participate in several local, state, and national projects including Girls on the Run, Adopt a Family, Relay for Life, WC SAFE, Angel House and Goodwill Inn Homeless Shelter.

Prerequisite Coursework

Human Anatomy, Human Physiology, Microbiology, Biochemistry, Developmental Psychology, Introductory Statistics. All courses must be completed by the fall semester of the application year.

MINNESOTA

AUGSBURG COLLEGE

Augsburg College
Email:
paprog@augsburg.edu

2211 Riverside Avenue
Campus Box 149
Minneapolis, MN 55454
Phone: 612-330-1399

Mission: The mission of the Augsburg College Physician Assistant Studies Program is based on a foundation of respect and sensitivity to persons of all cultures and backgrounds and oriented towards providing care to underserved populations. Students are well educated in current medical theory and practice, and graduates are encouraged to work in primary care settings. The program promotes dedication to excellence in performance, with the highest standards of ethics and integrity, and commitment to lifelong personal and professional development.

Accreditation:
Continued

Degree Offered:
Master (MSPAS)

Start Date: June annually

Program Length:
31 months

Class Capacity:
30 students

Tuition: $81,660

Seat Deposit: $500

CASPA Participant: Yes
Supplemental Application: Yes
Admissions: Not specified
Application Deadline: August 1

GPA Requirement:
Overall GPA 3.0; Science GPA 3.0
Healthcare Experience: Prefer 1000 hours, but not required. Experience with serving the underserved is preferred.
PA Shadowing: Preferred but not required.
Required Standardized Testing: None
Letters of Recommendation: Three required, no one specific required but they recommend that one letter be from an employer/colleague (a professional reference), one letter from a professor or adviser (an academic reference), and one from a person of your choice (i.e. someone you've worked with on underserved projects, volunteer experiences or in a health care setting)

No class data reported

Male: not reported
Female: not reported
Minority: not reported
GPA: not reported
Science GPA: not reported
GRE: not required
Faculty to Student Ratio: not reported
Average Healthcare Experience: not reported

PANCE Scores

5-year First Time Pass: 99%

Most Recent First Time Pass: 100%

Curriculum Structure

Didactic: 18 months
Clinical: 13 months
Rotations: 8 mandatory, 1 elective rotation; 1 preceptorship.
Capstone Course: Students present individual Master's research topic

Prerequisite Coursework

Developmental Psychology, Physiology, Microbiology, Biochemistry, General Statistics, Medical Terminology. Applicants can have prerequisites in progress at time of application.

Unique Program Features

Primary Care Focus: This program has a focus on providing primary care to the underserved populations. 72% of graduates report practicing in primary care after graduation, and many students continue to build on the community service begun prior to or during the PA program.

International Rotations: There are opportunities for students to complete international rotations and complete their Master's research project through an international experience.

Classes of 2016 and 2017

Male: 25%
Female: 75%
Minority: not reported
GPA: 3.73 (3.39-3.77 interquartile range)
Science GPA: 3.67 (3.24-3.67 interquartile range)
GRE: not required
Faculty to Student Ratio: not reported
Average Healthcare Experience: 1646 (330-59,000)

PANCE Scores

5-year First Time Pass: N/A (only one year of data available)

Most Recent First Time Pass: 100%

Curriculum Structure

Didactic: 15 months
Clinical: 12 months
Rotations: 7 mandatory, 2 elective rotation; Family Medicine and Internal Medicine are 8 weeks, all others are 4 weeks.
Evidence-Based Medicine/Thesis Project: Required for graduation

BETHEL UNIVERSITY

Bethel University
Email:
physician-assistant
@bethel.edu

3900 Bethel Drive
St. Paul, MN 55112
Phone: 651-635-8074

Mission: Boldly motivated by the Christian faith and in the spirit of Bethel University's academic excellence and ministry focus, the Bethel Physician Assistant program will educate students to become physician assistants who develop the skills for competent and excellent medical practice, live out ethical principles and Bethel's academic excellence, serve their community and all cultures, and possess integrity and compassion.

Accreditation:
Provisional

Degree Offered:
Master (MSPA)

Start Date:
June annually

Program Length:
27 months

Class Capacity:
32 students

Tuition: $82,880

GPA Requirement:
Overall GPA 3.25;
Science GPA 3.25;
Prerequisite GPA 3.25.

Healthcare Experience:
250 hours required.

PA Shadowing: Preferred, not required.

Required Standardized Testing: None

Letters of Recommendation: Two required, no one specific.

Seat Deposit: $500

CASPA Participant: Yes
Supplemental Application: Yes
Admissions: Not specified
Application Deadline: August 1

Prerequisite Coursework

Human Anatomy (3 credits), Human Physiology (3 credits), Organic Chemistry (3 credits), Biochemistry (3 credits), Microbiology (3 credits), Physics (3 credits), Psychology (3 credits), Statistics (3 credits). Applicants can have 3 prerequisites in progress at time of application.

Unique Program Features

Christian Tradition: The professors embrace a holistic approach to medical care that takes into account the mind, body, and spirit connection in medicine and how to integrate it with Christian faith in patient treatment.

Facilities: You will learn in a state-of-the-art training facility that uses patient simulators, video-monitored clinics, and other technologies to enhance learning.

ST. CATHERINE UNIVERSITY

Saint Catherine University

Email: mpas@stkate.edu

2004 Randolph Avenue #4027
Saint Paul, MN 55105
Phone: 651-690-6933

Mission: Influenced by Catholic intellectual tradition, the MPAS program is committed to preparing competent and compassionate Physician Assistant scholar practitioners who possess the knowledge, clinical acumen and critical thinking skills necessary to practice exemplary, ethical, patient-centered care, and who will lead and influence with grace emphasizing global responsibility, social justice and the preservation of human dignity.

Accreditation: Provisional

Degree Offered: Master (MPAS)

Start Date: September annually

Program Length: 28 months

Class Capacity: 32 students

Tuition: $80,960

CASPA Participant: Yes

Supplemental Application: No

Admissions: Non-rolling

Application Deadline: September 1

GPA Requirement: Overall GPA 3.2; Prerequisite GPA 3.0.

Healthcare Experience: Preferred, not required. Strongly encouraged to have a minimum of 250 hours.

PA Shadowing: Not required.

Required Standardized Testing: GRE

Letters of Recommendation: Two required, at least one recommendation should be from a healthcare provider; the other can be from a professor or employer.

Seat Deposit: $400

Class of 2017

Male: not reported
Female: not reported
Minority: not reported
GPA: 3.53
Prerequisite GPA: 3.5
GREVerbal: 156
GRE Quantitative: 155
GRE Writing: 4.0
Faculty to Student Ratio: not reported
Average Healthcare Experience: not reported

PANCE Scores

5-year First Time Pass: N/A (only one year of data available)

Most Recent First Time Pass: 100%

Curriculum Structure

Didactic: 14 months
Clinical: 14 months
Rotations: 7 mandatory, 2 elective rotation; ranging from 2-8 weeks in duration.

Professional Portfolio Presentation: Required for graduation

Prerequisite Coursework

Human or Vertebrate Anatomy (4 credits), Human or Vertebrate Physiology (4 credits), Organic Chemistry with Lab (8 credits), Biochemistry (3-4 credits), Microbiology (3-4 credits), Calculus (3-4 credits), Statistics (3-4 credits), Psychology (6 credits), Medical Terminology (1 course). At the time of application, no more than three courses may be in progress or yet to be taken.

Unique Program Features

International Experience: Students traveled for clinical rotation experience and medical mission trips to Haiti, Cuba, the Dominican Republic, South Korea, and Guatemala and participated in activities ranging from depression screenings to orthopedics care.

Curriculum Delivery: Though much of the content is delivered through lecture format, the program also focuses on small group clinical reasoning sessions and using educational technology throughout to enhance the student experience.

Inter-professional Education: There are opportunities for inter-professional education with nursing, occupational therapy, physical therapy and public health students within the Henrietta Schmoll School of Health.

MISSISSIPPI

MISSISSIPPI COLLEGE

Mississippi College
Email:
jrkendrick@mc.edu

Box 4053
Clinton, MS 39058
Phone: 601-925-7371

Mission: The primary mission of the Mississippi College Physician Assistant Program is to prepare physician assistants to provide primary health care services in medically underserved areas of Mississippi and surrounding states. Secondary missions are to prepare graduates for roles in surgery and as hospitalists.

Accreditation:
Continued

Degree Offered:
Master (MSM)

Start Date:
May annually

Program Length:
30 months

Class Capacity:
30 students

Tuition: $92,950

GPA Requirement:
Overall GPA 3.0;
Science GPA 3.0,
Prerequisite GPA 3.0

Healthcare Experience:
Preferred, not required

PA Shadowing: 1,000
hours recommended

Required Standardized Testing: GRE (minimum quantitative 140, verbal 146, and analytical 2.5)

Letters of Recommendation: Two required; no one specific.

Seat Deposit: $500

CASPA Participant: Yes

Supplemental Application: No

Admissions: Rolling

Application Deadline:
March 1

Class of 2017
Male: 47%
Female: 53%
Minority: 13%
GPA: 3.50
Science GPA: 3.42
GRE: not reported
Faculty to Student Ratio: not reported
Average Healthcare Experience:
2,600 hours

PANCE Scores

5-year First Time Pass:
92% (based on two years of data)

Most Recent First Time Pass: 97%

Curriculum Structure

Didactic: 16 months

Clinical: 12 months

Rotations:
7 mandatory,
1 elective, 1 advanced clerkship (12 weeks);
4 weeks each

Prerequisite Coursework

Human Anatomy and Physiology (8 credits), Microbiology (4 credits), General Chemistry (8 credits), Organic Chemistry (4 credits), Statistics (3 credits). You can have up to two prerequisites in progress at the time of application and all courses should be completed in the last 10 years.

Unique Program Features

Advanced Clerkship: This 12 week rotation allows students to choose one of three areas of concentration for their final semester of training (primary care, critical care, or surgery) and spend the entire semester at one training site.

Admissions Preference: The program gives preference to Mississippi residents.

MISSOURI

MISSOURI STATE UNIVERSITY

Missouri State University
Email:
PhysicianAsstStudies
@missouristate.edu

901 S. National Avenue
Springfield, MO 65897
Phone: not reported

Mission: The Missouri State University Physician Assistant Program seeks to prepare highly competent physician assistant graduates to practice primary care medicine in the context of team delivered care in a rapidly evolving health care arena. Using the resources of the College of Health and Human Services and affiliated clinical sites, the Program seeks to provide a comprehensive didactic and clinical educational experience for its students that incorporates the principles of scientific inquiry, self-directed study, critical analysis and problem-solving, all within the context of holistic care.

Accreditation:
Continued

Degree Offered:
Master (MSPAS)

Start Date:
May annually

Program Length:
24 months

Class Capacity:
32 students

Tuition:
In-state: $23,655;
Out-of-state: $44,903

GPA Requirement:
Overall GPA 3.0

Healthcare Experience:
500 hours

PA Shadowing: 24 hours preferred

Required Standardized Testing: GRE or MCAT

Letters of Recommendation: Three required; no one specific.

Seat Deposit: $500

CASPA Participant: Yes

Supplemental Application: No

Admissions: Not specified

Application Deadline: July 15

Class of 2016

Male: not reported
Female: not reported
Minority: not reported
GPA: 3.58
Science GPA: 3.51
GRE Combined: 301
Faculty to Student Ratio: not reported
Average Healthcare Experience: 5,219 hours

PANCE Scores

5-year First Time Pass: 92%

Most Recent First Time Pass: 90%

Curriculum Structure

Didactic: 12 months

Clinical: 12 months

Rotations: 7 mandatory, 1 elective; 6 weeks each

Research Paper: required for graduation

Prerequisite Coursework

Anatomy and Physiology with lab (8 credits), Microbiology (3 credits), Genetics (3 credits), General Chemistry (8 credits), Organic Chemistry of Biochemistry (4 credits), Statistics (3 credits), General or Introductory Psychology (3 credits), Social Science (3 credits). They prefer that applicants complete courses within the last five years.

Unique Program Features

Underserved Populations: All students are required to do at least one underserved or rural population rotation.

Admissions Preference: The program has a preference for Missouri residents.

Facilities: The O'Reilly Clinical Health Science Center was completed in 2015 and houses the PA program. It includes a large classroom, laboratory for clinical skills training, state-of-the-art clinical simulation facility, and dedicated graduate student study areas.

Class of 2017

Male: 17%

Female: 83%

Minority: not reported

GPA: 3.70

Science GPA: 3.65

GRE Combined: not required

Faculty to Student Ratio: not reported

Average Healthcare Experience: 4,150 hours

PANCE Scores

5-year First Time Pass: 99%

Most Recent First Time Pass: 100%

Curriculum Structure

Didactic: 15 months

Clinical: 12 months

Rotations: 8 mandatory, 2 elective, 4-6 weeks each

Saint Louis University Physician Assistant Education Department

3437 Caroline Street
Saint Louis, MO 63104
Phone: 314-977-8521
Email: paprog@slu.edu

Mission: The primary mission of the Saint Louis University Physician Assistant Program is to educate men and women to become competent, compassionate physician assistants dedicated to excellence in healthcare and the service of humanity.

Accreditation: Continued

Degree Offered: Master (MMS)

Start Date: August annually

Program Length: 27 months

Class Capacity: 34 students

Tuition: $77.055

GPA Requirement: Overall GPA 3.0; Science GPA 3.0

Healthcare Experience: 500 hours

PA Shadowing: Recommended, not required

Required Standardized Testing: None

Letters of Recommendation: Three required; no one specific.

Seat Deposit: $850

CASPA Participant: Yes

Supplemental Application: Yes

Admissions: Rolling

Application Deadline: November 1

Unique Program Features

Community Service: There is a 12 hour minimum of community service for all students in the program which can include shopping for an elderly neighbor, tending to children in respite care and assisting at community health fairs to organized events like Make a Difference Day, the Open Doors Event and SLU's Campus Kitchen.

Student Clinic: All students also volunteer in the student-operated free health clinic which includes days for adults, pediatrics, women, cardiology, diabetes, asthma, allergy, and homeless patients.

Prerequisite Coursework

Medical Terminology (1-3 credits), Statistics (3 credits), Chemistry I and II (8 credits), Organic Chemistry I and II (6-8 credits), Microbiology (3-4 credits), Vertebrate or Human Anatomy (3-4 credits), Vertebrate or Human Physiology (3-4 credits), Genetics (3-4 credits). Courses may be in progress at time of application and should be completed within seven years of application.

UNIVERSITY OF MISSOURI – KANSAS CITY

University of Missouri - Kansas City
Email: medicine@umkc.edu

2411 Holmes Street
M1-103
Kansas City, MO 64108
Phone: 816-235-1870

Mission: To educate competent, compassionate, and culturally-aware Physician Assistants who are prepared to meet the healthcare needs of our community. Graduates will advance the Physician Assistant profession through clinical excellence, service, and dedication to lifelong learning.

Accreditation:
Provisional

Degree Offered:
Master (MMS)

Start Date:
January annually

Program Length:
29 months

Class Capacity:
20 students

Tuition:
In-state: $69,556;
Out-of-state: $82,678

GPA Requirement:
Overall GPA 3.0;
Prerequisite GPA 3.0

Healthcare Experience:
Preferred, not required

PA Shadowing: 8 hours required

Required Standardized Testing: GRE or MCAT

Letters of Recommendation: Three required; no one specific.

Seat Deposit: $300

CASPA Participant: Yes

Supplemental Application: Yes

Admissions: Non-rolling

Application Deadline:
August 1

Prerequisite Coursework

Biology with lab, Anatomy with lab, Physiology with lab, Microbiology with lab, General Chemistry I and II with lab, Organic Chemistry with lab, Biochemistry, Statistics, Medical Terminology. Two courses can be incomplete at the time of application and it is preferred that all courses be completed within seven years of the application deadline.

No class statistics reported

PANCE Scores
5-year First Time Pass: N/A

Most Recent First Time Pass: N/A (have not graduated a class yet)

Curriculum Structure
Didactic: 17 months

Clinical: 12 months

Rotations:
10 mandatory,
2 elective,
4 weeks each

Capstone Project:
required for graduation

Unique Program Features

Admissions Preference: Missouri residents are preferred in the admissions process with the goal of 80% of each class being from Missouri.

Student Profiles: Profiles of current students are available on the website to get an insider perspective on the program.

MONTANA

ROCKY MOUNTAIN COLLEGE

Rocky Mountain
College
Email: PA@rocky.edu

1511 Poly Drive
Billings, MT 59102
Phone: 406-657-1190

PANCE Scores

5-year First Time Pass:
98%

Most Recent First Time
Pass: 100%

Curriculum Structure

Didactic: 14 months

Clinical: 12 months

Rotations:
7 mandatory,
1 elective,
6 weeks each

Capstone Project:
required for
graduation

Unique Program Features

*Admissions
Preference:* Applicants
from Montana, Wyoming,
Colorado, North Dakota,
South Dakota, Utah
or Idaho are given
preference points in the
admissions profess as
are those who graduated
high school in a rural
area.

Mission: The mission of the Master of Physician Assistant Studies Program (MPAS) is to provide a quality medical education, which integrates academic training with the development of essential clinical skills and professionalism. We seek to graduate individuals who are intellectually engaged, analytical, and are committed to providing compassionate health care services, particularly to those in rural and underserved areas of this region.

Accreditation:
Continued

Degree Offered:
Master (MPAS)

Start Date:
July annually

Program Length:
26 months

Class Capacity:
36 students

Tuition:
$97,850 (fees included)

GPA Requirement:
Overall GPA 3.0;
Science GPA 2.7

Healthcare Experience:
1500 hours required

PA Shadowing:
not required

*Required Standardized
Testing:* GRE (minimum
score 291)

*Letters of
Recommendation:* Three
required; no one specific.

Seat Deposit: $1,000

CASPA Participant: Yes

*Supplemental
Application:* No

Admissions: Rolling

Application Deadline:
October 1

Prerequisite Coursework

Human Anatomy and Physiology with lab (8 credits), Microbiology with lab (4 credits), Genetics (3 credits), Medical Terminology (1-2 credits), Mathematics (3 credits), Statistics (3 credits), Psychology (3 credits), Social Science (3 credits), English Composition (3 credits), General or Organic or Biochemistry (1 year sequence).

NEBRASKA

UNIVERSITY OF NEBRASKA

University of Nebraska
Email:
sahpadmissions
@unmc.edu

984035 Nebraska Medical
Center
Omaha, NE 68198-4035
Phone: 402-559-6673

Mission: The mission of the Physician Assistant Program at the University of Nebraska Medical Center is to educate a diverse student population as entry-level practitioners of primary care medicine, working with physician supervision, in order to provide the citizens of Nebraska, particularly those in rural and underserved areas, with quality medical care.

Accreditation:
Continued

Degree Offered:
Master (MPAS)

Start Date:
August annually

Program Length:
28 months

Class Capacity:
58 students

Tuition:
In-state: $31,610;
Out-of-state: $90,443

GPA Requirement:
Overall GPA 3.0

Healthcare Experience:
Preferred, not required

PA Shadowing:
Not required

Required Standardized Testing: GRE

Letters of Recommendation: Three required; one academic letter and one from a health professional. No friend or family references

Seat Deposit: $500

CASPA Participant: Yes
Supplemental Application: No

Admissions: Not specified
Application Deadline:
September 1

Class of 2015
Male: 19%
Female: 81%
Minority:
not reported
GPA: 3.80 (3.52-3.99)
Science GPA:
3.71 (3.19-4.0)
GRE Verbal: 154
GRE Quantitative:
155
GRE Writing: 4.0
Faculty to Student Ratio: not reported
Average Healthcare Experience:
not reported

PANCE Scores

5-year First Time Pass:
98%

Most Recent First Time Pass: 100%

Curriculum Structure

Didactic: 13 months
Clinical: 15 months
Rotations:
8 mandatory,
5 electives; 4 weeks each except 12 weeks of family medicine.

Prerequisite Coursework

Biology (4 credits), Human Anatomy (4 credits), Human Physiology (4 credits), Microbiology (4 credits), General or Inorganic Chemistry (8 credits), Organic Chemistry with lab (4 credits), Biochemistry (4 credits), General Psychology (3 credits), Abnormal Psychology (3 credits), Life Span/Developmental Psychology or other elective (3 credits), Statistics (3 credits), English Composition (3 credits), Additional Writing or English Composition (3 credits). Courses can be in progress at time of application.

Unique Program Features

Two Campuses: This program operates with 58 students total split between the University of Nebraska Medical Center at Omaha and University of Nebraska Kearney Campuses.

Admissions Preference: The admissions committee gives preference to applicants with an overall and science GPA of 3.20 or greater, GRE scores at 50th percentile or greater, those with strong motivation to practice in medically underserved area, prior work or volunteer direct patient care, significant extracurricular, professional, or service organization activity, and Nebraska residents.

Dual Degree: A dual PA/MPH program is offered with a specialization in Community-Oriented Primary Care within the Department of Health Promotion and takes just over three years to complete.

UNION COLLEGE

No class statistics reported

PANCE Scores

5-year First Time Pass: 91%

Most Recent First Time Pass: 93%

Curriculum Structure

Didactic: 21 months

Clinical: 12 months

Rotations: 10 mandatory, 1 elective; 4 weeks each.

Capstone Project: Required for graduation

Unique Program Features

Christian Influence: This school has a Seventh-day Adventist heritage and students must adhere to a lifestyle agreement dedicated to the high ethical and moral values of Christian living as a condition for acceptance at the program.

Early Clinical Exposure: Students begin helping patients early in the curriculum through volunteering at foot clinics, community kitchens, and other outreach programs.

Union College
Email: paprog@ucollege.edu

3800 South 48th Street
Lincoln, NE 68506-4386
Phone: 402-486-2527

Mission: The Union College Physician Assistant Program prepares students from diverse backgrounds for excellence in the Physician Assistant profession, developing their God-given abilities in harmony with the highest physical, mental, social and spiritual ideals.

Accreditation: Continued

Degree Offered: Master (MPAS)

Start Date: August annually

Program Length: 33 months

Class Capacity: 30 students

Tuition: $98,016 (tuition + fees)

Seat Deposit: $650

GPA Requirement: Overall GPA 2.8; Science GPA 2.8

Healthcare Experience: 480 hours required, at least 240 completed by time of application

PA Shadowing: Required

Required Standardized Testing: Not required

Letters of Recommendation: Three required; It is recommended that one letter come from an employer, one letter from a professor, and one from someone who knows your character (i.e. clergyman)

CASPA Participant: Yes

Supplemental Application: No

Admissions: Not specified

Application Deadline: October 1

Prerequisite Coursework

General Biology with labs (8 credits), Microbiology with lab (4 credits), Anatomy with lab (4 credits), Physiology with lab (4 credits), General/Organic Chemistry (8-16 credits), Biochemistry with lab preferred (3-4 credits), Medical Terminology (1 credit), Elementary Statistics and Probability (3 credits), Developmental (Lifespan) Psychology (3 credits), AHA Healthcare Provider CPR. Generally science courses should be completed in the last 7 years.

NEVADA

TOURO UNIVERSITY NEVADA

Touro University
Email:
admissions@tun.touro.edu

874 American Pacific Drive
Henderson, NV 89014
Phone: 702-777-8687

Mission: The Master of Physician Assistant Studies Program is committed to the education of highly qualified compassionate Physician Assistants who are part of the health care team and are responsive to the developing health needs of their communities as culturally competent clinicians, educators, facilitators, and leaders.

Accreditation:
Continued

Degree Offered:
Master (MPAS)

Start Date:
July annually

Program Length:
28 months

Class Capacity:
60 students

Tuition:
$83,000 (approximate)

GPA Requirement: Overall GPA 2.75; Science GPA 2.75

Healthcare Experience:
Preferred, not required

PA Shadowing:
not required

Required Standardized Testing: None

Letters of Recommendation: Three required; no one specific.

Seat Deposit: $1,000

CASPA Participant: Yes

Supplemental Application: Yes

Admissions: Rolling

Application Deadline:
September 1

Prerequisite Coursework

Human Anatomy and Physiology (8 credits), Inorganic Chemistry (4 credits), Organic Chemistry (4 credits), Biochemistry (3 credits), Microbiology (3 credits). All courses must be completed at the time of the application and all courses should be completed in the last five years except organic and inorganic chemistry.

PANCE Scores

5-year First Time Pass: 93%

Most Recent First Time Pass: 93%

Curriculum Structure

Didactic: 16 months

Clinical: 12 months

Rotations:
8 mandatory,
2 elective,
4-8 weeks each

Unique Program Features

Inter-professional Education: As the program is offered on campus with osteopathy, physical therapy, and nursing students, PA program students learn to work with all health care team members and also complete a service-learning course that prepares graduates to be culturally sensitive and advocates for the community.

NEW HAMPSHIRE

FRANKLIN PIERCE

Franklin Pierce University
Email: paprogram @franklinpierce.edu

24 Airport Road
West Lebanon, NH 03784
Phone: 603-298-6617

Mission: The mission of the Franklin Pierce University Physician Assistant Program is to graduate competent and compassionate physician assistants who possess the requisite knowledge, skills, and attitudes to provide high quality, patient-oriented primary care in diverse environments.

Accreditation:
Continuing

Degree Offered:
Master (MPAS)

Start Date:
November annually

Program Length:
27 months

Class Capacity:
24 students

Tuition: $88,722

GPA Requirement:
Overall GPA 2.8;
Science GPA 3.0

Healthcare Experience:
Preferred/Recommended

PA Shadowing:
Required (20 hours)

Required Standardized Testing: Not required

Letters of Recommendation: Three required; not from anyone specific

Seat Deposit: $500

CASPA Participant: Yes

Supplemental Application: Yes

Admissions: Rolling

Application Deadline:
November 1

Prerequisite Coursework

Anatomy and Physiology with lab (2 semesters), Chemistry with lab (2 semesters), Biology with lab (1 semester)

Microbiology with lab (1 semester), Statistics (1 semester), Psychology (1 semester).Up to two prerequisites may be outstanding at the time of application, but these must be completed with a grade of "B" or better.

Class Statistics
GPA: 3.5
Science GPA: 3.5

PANCE Scores

5-year First Time Pass: 91% (based on 4 years of scores)

Most Recent First Time Pass: 86%

Curriculum Structure

Didactic: 12 months
Clinical: 15 months
Rotations:
8 mandatory (5 weeks long), 1 elective (4 weeks long)

Project: Case presentation and community service project required for graduation

Unique Program Features

Student Demographic: The program strives to accept 40-50% of each class from applicants residing in NH/VT.

NEW JERSEY

MONMOUTH UNIVERSITY

Monmouth University
Graduate Admissions
Email:
paprogram@monmouth.edu

400 Cedar Avenue
West Long Branch, NJ 07764
Phone: 732-923-4505

Mission: The mission of the Monmouth University Physician Assistant Program is to educate physician assistants to provide compassionate, patient-centered quality health care in a variety of settings. Program graduates will possess clinical skills to serve a diverse patient population and have the ability to advance the profession through leadership and research.

Accreditation:
Provisional

Degree Offered:
Master (MS)

Start Date:
September annually

Program Length:
36 months (with summers off)

Class Capacity:
30 students

Tuition: $99,465

GPA Requirement:
Overall GPA 3.0;
Prerequisite GPA 3.0

Healthcare Experience: 200 hours required (200 hours)— Paid or volunteer experience with hands-on patient care

PA Shadowing: No specific requirement but shadowing hours can be counted towards healthcare experience.

Required Standardized Testing: GRE

Letters of Recommendation: Three required; not from anyone specific

Seat Deposit: $350

CASPA Participant: Yes

Supplemental Application: No

Admissions: Not reported

Application Deadline:
January 15

No class statistics reported

PANCE Scores
No scores available yet

Curriculum Structure
Didactic: 10 months
Clinical: 14 months
Rotations: 4 clinical clerkship blocks; no other details reported
Capstone Project: Not reported

Unique Program Features
Scholarship: Graduate Scholarships are offered by the University to students on the basis of their undergraduate GPA. Award values range from $2,400 to $5,100 per semester.

Location: Classes held at a satellite campus with classrooms and clinical skills laboratories dedicated for PA student use.

Prerequisite Coursework

Human Anatomy with lab (1 semester), Human Physiology with lab (1 semester), Chemistry I and II with lab (2 semesters), Biology I with lab (1 semester), Microbiology with lab (1 semester), General Psychology (1 semester), Medical Terminology (1 course, 1-3 credits), Math (either Pre-calculus, Calculus, or Statistics) (1 semester)

Class of 2018

GPA: 3.66
Science GPA: 3.61

PANCE Scores

5-year First Time Pass: 98%

Most Recent First Time Pass: 100%

Curriculum Structure

Didactic: 16 months

Clinical: 17 months

Rotations: 9 mandatory, 2 elective (range from 3-8 weeks)

Capstone Project: Evidence-based literature review required for graduation

Unique Program Features

Program: Offers a combined BA/MS track through one of their affiliated universities (see website for qualifying schools). A part-time curriculum is also available and interested students should contact the PA program for details.

Joint MS/MPH: Students can earn a joint degree in four years (including summers).

RUTGERS UNIVERSITY

Rutgers University
Email: pa-info@shrp.rutgers.edu

675 Hoes Lane West
Piscataway, NJ 08854-5635
Phone: 732-235-4445

Mission: The Rutgers University Physician Assistant Program enhances the delivery of humanistic patient care and advances the PA profession through a dynamic blend of educational programs research and service. Expertly crafted curricula and thoughtful mentorship of students develop collaborative, caring and competent health care providers.

Accreditation: Continuing

Degree Offered: Master (MS)

Start Date: August annually

Program Length: 33 months

Class Capacity: 50 students

Tuition: $19,260/year for in-state students and $28,890/year for out-of-state students

CASPA Participant: Yes

Supplemental Application: Yes

Admissions: Rolling

Application Deadline: September 1

GPA Requirement: Overall GPA 3.2; Science GPA 3.2

Healthcare Experience: Required (no specific number of hours)—Paid or volunteer experience with hands-on patient care

PA Shadowing: Required (no specific number of hours)

Required Standardized Testing: None

Letters of Recommendation: Three required; Applicants should seek recommendations from individuals who are thoroughly familiar with the candidate's academic ability, their work ethic and professionalism, and their general characteristics.

Seat Deposit: $500

Prerequisite Coursework

Biological Sciences with lab (2 semesters), General Chemistry with lab (2 semesters), Organic Chemistry (1 semester), General Psychology (1 semester), English Composition (1 semester), Statistics (preferably Applied Statistics or Biostatistics from the Psychology, Biology or Math Dept.) (1 semester)

SETON HALL

Seton Hall University
Email: physician-assistant@shu.edu

400 South Orange Avenue
South Orange, NJ 7079
Phone: 973-275-2596

Mission: The mission of the Physician Assistant (PA) program at Seton Hall University is to prepare primary care PAs who practice in diverse settings. The program provides the foundation for graduates to become critical thinkers who practice evidence-based, patient-centered medicine.

Accreditation:
Continuing

Degree Offered:
Master of Science

Start Date:
August annually

Program Length:
33 months (summers off)

Class Capacity:
34 students

Tuition: $108,960

GPA Requirement:
Overall GPA 3.2;
Prerequisite GPA 3.2

Healthcare Experience:
100 hours required

PA Shadowing: No specific number of hours; can be counted toward healthcare experience

Required Standardized Testing: GRE

Letters of Recommendation: Three required; not from anyone specific

Seat Deposit: $500

CASPA Participant: No

Supplemental Application: Yes

Admissions:

Application Deadline:
December 15

No class statistics reported

PANCE Scores
5-year First Time Pass: 99%

Most Recent First Time Pass: 96%

Curriculum Structure
Didactic: 12 months

Clinical: 15 months

Rotations:
9 mandatory (ranging from 4-12 weeks), 1 elective (4 weeks)

Capstone Project:
Group research project required for graduation

Unique Program Features
None provided

Prerequisite Coursework

General Biology I and II with lab (2 semesters), Chemistry I and II with lab (2 semesters), Anatomy and Physiology I and II with lab (2 semesters), Microbiology with lab (1 semester), Psychology (1 semester), Math (Pre-calculus, calculus, statistics) (1 semester)

NEW MEXICO

UNIVERSITY OF NEW MEXICO

University of New Mexico

Email: paprogram@salud.unm.edu

MSC09 5040
1 University of New Mexico
Albuquerque, NM 87131-0000
Phone: 505-272-9864

Mission: The mission of the University of New Mexico Physician Assistant Program is to educate Physician Assistant students to be competent providers of primary care medicine, with a special focus on the medically under-served and/or rural populations of New Mexico.

Accreditation:
Continued

Degree Offered:
Master (MSPAS)

Start Date:
June annually

Program Length:
27 months

Class Capacity:
17 students

Tuition:
In-state: $48,157;
Out-of-state: $71,181

GPA Requirement:
Overall GPA 3.0;
Science GPA 3.0;
Prerequisite GPA 2.0

Healthcare Experience:
500 hours required

PA Shadowing:
Preferred, not required

Required Standardized Testing: GRE

Letters of Recommendation: Three required; One from a PA-C, physician, or DO

Seat Deposit: $250

CASPA Participant: Yes

Supplemental Application: Yes

Admissions: Not specified

Application Deadline:
August 1

Class of 2017
Male: 35%
Female: 65%
Minority: 59%
GPA: 3.74
Science GPA: 3.70
GRE Quantitative: 153
GRE Verbal: 147
GRE Analytical: 3.9
Faculty to Student Ratio: not reported
Average Healthcare Experience: 5,446 hours

PANCE Scores
5-year First Time Pass: 92%

Most Recent First Time Pass: 94%

Curriculum Structure
Didactic: 15 months
Clinical: 12 months
Rotations: 8 mandatory, 1 elective, 4-6 weeks each

Prerequisite Coursework

General Biology with lab (4 credits), General Chemistry I and II with lab (8 credits) Human Anatomy and Physiology I and II with lab (8 credits), Psychology (3 credits), Statistics (3 credits), English (6 credits). Science courses must have been taken in the last 10 years.

Unique Program Features

Problem Based Learning: On average six hours per week are devoted to problem based learning in small groups where students are exposed to pathophysiology, behavioral medicine, and population health.

Admissions Preference: The program prefers applicants who are residents of New Mexico. All students from the class of 2017 were New Mexico residents.

Class of 2017

Male: not reported
Female: not reported
Minority: not reported
GPA: 3.49
Science GPA: 3.37
GRE: not reported
Faculty to Student Ratio: not reported
Average Healthcare Experience: 1,200 hours

PANCE Scores

5-year First Time Pass: 94%

Most Recent First Time Pass: 100%

Curriculum Structure

Didactic: 15 months
Clinical: 12 months
Rotations: 7 mandatory, 1 elective, 6 weeks each

Unique Program Features

Rural Focus: All students must complete at least two rural rotations during the clinical year.

Community Service: Faculty and students participate in community service together throughout the program. Recent projects have included food banks, 5k runs, a teddy bear drive, nursing home visits, school supply drives, care packages, and providing Christmas presents to underprivileged kids.

University of St. Francis
Email: rvigil@stfrancis.edu

1500 N. Renaissance NE
Suite C
Albuquerque, NM 87107
Phone: 505-266-5565

Mission: The mission of the PA program is to educate highly qualified Physician Assistants preparing them to become competent, compassionate and comprehensive health care providers for practice in medically underserved areas.

Accreditation: Continued

Degree Offered: Master (MSPAS)

Start Date: January annually

Program Length: 27 months

Class Capacity: 30 students

Tuition: $68,850

GPA Requirement: Overall GPA 3.0; Science GPA 3.0; Prerequisite GPA 3.0

Healthcare Experience: 250 hours required

PA Shadowing: not required

Required Standardized Testing: GRE

Letters of Recommendation: Three required; no one specific

Seat Deposit: $500

CASPA Participant: Yes
Supplemental Application: No

Admissions: Not specified
Application Deadline: November 1

Prerequisite Coursework

General Biology I with lab, General Biology II with lab or Cell and Molecular Biology, Anatomy with lab, Physiology, General Chemistry I and II with lab, Statistics, Genetics, Microbiology. All prerequisites must be taken within five years of admission to the program and should be completed prior to application.

NEWYORK

ALBANY MEDICAL COLLEGE

Center for Physician Assistant Studies
Albany Medical College

47 New Scotland Ave. MC-4
Albany, NY 12208-3412
Phone:518-262-5251
Email:greenr@mail.amc.edu

Mission: The Center for Physician Assistant Studies, In support of Albany Medical Center's mission as an academic health sciences center, has a responsibility to educate Physician Assistant students from demographically diverse backgrounds to meet the future primary and specialty health care needs of the region and the country by providing highly skilled, cost-effective, patient-centered care in a variety of settings. This mission will be advanced through commitment to the values of Quality and Excellence, Collaboration, Confidentiality, Respect and Compassion, Integrity, Responsibility, Diversity, and Community Service.

Accreditation:
Continuing

Degree Offered:
Master (MSPAS)

Start Date:
January annually

Program Length:
28 months

Class Capacity:
42 students

Tuition: $55,272

GPA Requirement:
No minimum

Healthcare Experience:
1000 hours required

PA Shadowing:
Not reported

Required Standardized Testing: GRE

Letters of Recommendation: Three required; not from anyone specific

Seat Deposit: $500

CASPA Participant: Yes

Supplemental Application: Yes

Admissions: Rolling

Application Deadline:
December 1

Prerequisite Coursework

General Biology with lab (2 semesters), General Chemistry with lab (2 semesters), Biochemistry, Organic Chemistry or other advanced chemistry (1 semester), Anatomy and Physiology with lab (2 semesters), Microbiology with lab (1 semester), Psychology (1 semester), Statistics (1 semester), English Composition (1 semester)

Class Demographics Class of 2017

Male: Not reported

Female: Not reported

Minority: Not reported

GPA: 3.55

Science GPA: 3.46

GRE:
Verbal – 62%;
Quantitative – 58%;
Analytical – 54%

Faculty to Student Ratio: Not reported

Average Healthcare Experience: 2,979 hours

PANCE Scores

5-year First Time Pass: 96%

Most Recent First Time Pass: 97%

Curriculum Structure

Didactic: 16 months

Clinical: 12 months

Rotations:
10 mandatory, 2 electives

Portfolio Project:
Required for graduation

Unique Program Features

*Reputation:*Among the oldest PA Programs in the nation (42 years) and continuously accredited since 1972.

PANCE Scores

5-year First Time Pass: 95%

Most Recent First Time Pass: 97%

Curriculum Structure

Didactic: 13 months

Clinical: 13 months

Rotations: 9 mandatory (seven are 6 weeks long, two are 4 weeks long), 1 elective (4 weeks long)

Research Methods Project: Required for graduation

Unique Program Features

Diversity: The Physician Assistant Program is committed to increasing the number of physician assistants of African-American, Latino, and other ethnic backgrounds, whose communities have historically been underserved.

CCNY SOPHIE DAVIS SCHOOL OF BIOMEDICAL EDUCATION

CCNY Sophie Davis School of BiomedicalEducation

PA Admissions Committee

160 Convent Avenue
Harris Hall-15
New York, NY 10031
Phone: 212-650-7745
Email: paprogadmissions @med.cuny.edu

Mission: The mission of the SDSBE Physician Assistant Program is to improve the health of underserved communities and to eliminate healthcare disparity by providing increased access to physician assistant education to students from traditionally underrepresented populations. Through education and mentoring, we will create a workforce that will provide highly skilled primary health services to the communities of greatest need.

Accreditation: Continuing

Degree Offered: Master (MSPAS)

Start Date: August annually

Program Length: 28.5 months

Class Capacity: 35 students

Tuition: $35,455 (in-state); $62,400 (out-of-state)

GPA Requirement: Overall GPA 3.0; Prerequisite GPA 3.0

Healthcare Experience: Preferred/Recommended

PA Shadowing: Not reported

Required Standardized Testing: None

Letters of Recommendation: Three required; one should be from a physician or physician assistant who can attest, from first-hand experience, any abilities the applicant will bring to the profession

Seat Deposit: $650

CASPA Participant: Yes

Supplemental Application: Yes

Admissions: Not reported

Application Deadline: January 15

Prerequisite Coursework

Biology with lab (2 semesters), Chemistry with lab (2 semesters), Microbiology with lab (1 semester), Statistics (1 semester), Two of the following: Cell and Molecular Biology, Genetics, Mammalian Physiology, Anatomy and Physiology with lab (2 semesters), Biochemistry

All prerequisites must be completed with a grade of "C" or better. Up to two prerequisite courses may be pending when the application is submitted, as long as they will be completed by June 1st.

CLARKSON UNIVERSITY

Clarkson University
Department of
Physician Assistant
Studies

8 Clarkson Avenue
Box 5882
Potsdam, NY 13699-5882
Phone:315-268-7942
Email: pa@clarkson.edu

Mission: The mission of the Clarkson University Department of Physician Assistant Studies is to educate Physician Assistants to become highly skilled and compassionate health care providers. The program will encourage an interdisciplinary approach with an emphasis on patient-centered care.

Accreditation:
Continuing

Degree Offered:
Master (MSPAS)

Start Date:
January annually

Program Length:
28 months

Class Capacity:
30 students

Tuition:
$14,460 per semester
(no total given)

GPA Requirement:
Overall GPA 3.0; Science GPA; Prerequisite GPA 3.0

Healthcare Experience:
500 hours required

PA Shadowing: Required (at least 1 day)—a form will need to be filled out by the PA you shadow

Required Standardized Testing: GRE

Letters of Recommendation:
Three required; One from a MD, PA or NP

Seat Deposit: $1,000

CASPA Participant: Yes

Supplemental Application: Yes

Admissions: Rolling

Application Deadline:
March 1

Prerequisite Coursework

Biology (2 semesters), Anatomy and Physiology (2 semesters), Microbiology (can fulfill the requirement for one of the two Biology courses needed), Chemistry (2 semesters; Organic Chemistry is recommended), Social Sciences/Humanities (1 semester), Statistics (1 semester), Genetics (1 semester), Psychology (1 semester)

Courses must be complete or in progress at the time of application.

No class statistics reported

PANCE Scores

5-year First Time Pass: 100% (based on only two years of scores)

Most Recent First Time Pass: 100%

Curriculum Structure

Didactic: 13 months

Clinical: 14 months + 1 summative month

Rotations:
7 mandatory, 2 elective, 1 clinical research elective (all 5 weeks long)

Master's Project:
Required for graduation

Unique Program Features

Pre-PA: The school offers a pre-PA plan for undergraduates entering Clarkson with an interest in pursuing a career as a PA. Ten seats in each cohort are held for Clarkson pre-PA students.

Community Service: Service has been an integral part of our student's experience. Our students have volunteered for our local Hospice, Food Bank, Christmas Fund, Office of the Aging, blood pressure screenings, Relay for Life, and a Red Cross blood drive. Many students went on a mission trip to the Dominican Republic with plans in place to continue yearly missions.

PANCE Scores

5-year First Time Pass: 93%

Most Recent First Time Pass: 100%

Curriculum Structure

Didactic: 10 months

Clinical: 16 months

Rotations: 10 mandatory, 5 electives

Project: A scholarly literature review and research proposal and defense are both required for graduation

Unique Program Features

Surgical Focus: The program has a focus on surgery in didactic and clinical curricula though all aspects of primary care are covered as well for the PANCE.

CORNELL UNIVERSITY

Cornell University
Email: mshspa@med.cornell.edu

575 Lexington Avenue
Suite 600
New York, NY 10022
Phone: 646-962-7277

Mission: The principal mission of the Weill Cornell Medical College Physician Assistant Program is to educate highly competent, safe and effective physician assistants capable of practicing and excelling in diverse clinical and academic settings. The Program offers a rigorous and thorough foundation in generalist medicine and primary care education, striving for a balanced curriculum that provides students with fundamental principles of generalist clinical practice and training in general surgery and the surgical subspecialties. Consistent with the mission of its sponsoring institution, the program will develop a course of study and scholarship, which will allow its students to obtain a Masters degree in Health Science. In this way, the program will advance medical knowledge and contribute to the PA profession through research and other scholarly endeavors.

Accreditation: Continuing

Degree Offered: Master (MHS)

Start Date: March annually

Program Length: 26 months

Class Capacity: 32 students

Tuition: $76,482

GPA Requirement: 3.0 overall GPA

Healthcare Experience: 200 hours required

PA Shadowing: Strongly recommended

Required Standardized Testing: GRE

Letters of Recommendation: Two required; One from a physician or PA and one from a prior professor or instructor

Seat Deposit: $700

CASPA Participant: Yes

Supplemental Application: Yes

Admissions: Not reported

Application Deadline: September 1

Prerequisite Coursework

Biology with lab (2 semesters), Chemistry with lab (2 semesters), Microbiology (1 semester), Biochemistry (1 semester), Anatomy and Physiology (2 semesters)
English Composition (1 semester)

CUNY YORK

CUNY York College
Email:
paprogram
@york.cuny.edu

94-20 Guy R. Brewster Boulevard
Science Building Room SC-112
Jamaica, NY 11451
Phone:718-262-2823

Mission: The York College Physician Assistant program seeks to recruit and educate students from the diverse surrounding communities to become highly competent, compassionate, and culturally aware providers of excellent medical care to underserved urban areas. Incorporated in our mission is a priority on increasing access to medical professional education for racial and ethnic minorities, financially disadvantaged students, and first-generation college graduates. Our program is committed to providing strong supports so that we may also expect high performance from our students.

Accreditation:
Continuing

Degree Offered:
Master (MSPAS)

Start Date:
August annually

Program Length:
24 months

Class Capacity:
60 students

Tuition:
$5,065 per semester
(in-state);
$36,660 total
(out-of-state)

GPA Requirement:
Overall GPA 3.0;
Science GPA 3.0

Healthcare Experience:
200 hours

PA Shadowing: Can be counted towards healthcare experience hours

Required Standardized Testing: GRE

Letters of Recommendation:
Three required; not from anyone specific

Seat Deposit: None

CASPA Participant: Yes

Supplemental Application: No

Admissions: Not reported

Application Deadline:
January 15

No class statistics reported

PANCE Scores

5-year First Time Pass:
80%

Most Recent First Time Pass: 89%

Curriculum Structure

Didactic: 12 months

Clinical: 12 months

Rotations:
9 mandatory (each 5 weeks long)

Capstone Project:
Not required

Unique Program Features

None reported

Prerequisite Coursework

General Biology (2 semesters), General Chemistry (2 semesters), Biochemistry (1 semester), Human Anatomy and Physiology (2 semesters), Microbiology (1 semester), Statistics (1 semester), Behavior Science such as Psychology, Sociology or Anthropology (2 semesters)

Class Statistics

Male: Not reported

Female: Not reported

Minority: Not reported

GPA: 3.5

Science GPA: 3.4

GRE: Not required

Faculty to Student Ratio: Not reported

Average Healthcare Experience: Not reported

PANCE Scores

5-year First Time Pass: 98%

Most Recent First Time Pass: 100%

Curriculum Structure

Didactic: 18 months

Clinical: 15 months

Rotations: 10 mandatory (each 4 weeks long)

Research Project: Required for graduation

Unique Program Features

Community Service: The program founded Students Without Borders and makes an annual mission trip to the Dominican Republic.

Daemen College
Email: vsanlore@daemen.edu

Curtis Hall
4380 Main Street
Amherst, NY 14226
Phone: 716-839-8383

Mission: The mission of the Daemen College Physician Assistant Program is to educate capable individuals to meet the challenges of providing quality health care services with the supervision of a licensed physician.

Accreditation: Continuing

Degree Offered: MS; combined BS/MS available as well

Start Date: September annually

Program Length: 33 months

Class Capacity: 65 students (20-25 seats available for graduate applicants)

Tuition: $100,568

GPA Requirement: Overall GPA 3.0; Science GPA 3.0; Prerequisite GPA 3.0

Healthcare Experience: 120 hours required

PA Shadowing: Counts towards healthcare experience hours

Required Standardized Testing: None

Letters of Recommendation: Three required; not from anyone specific

Seat Deposit: $500

CASPA Participant: Yes

Supplemental Application: Yes

Admissions: Not reported

Application Deadline: January 15

Prerequisite Coursework

Biology with lab (2 semesters), General Chemistry (2 semesters), Calculus (1 semester), Psychology and/or Sociology (3 semesters), Anatomy and Physiology with lab (2 semesters), Microbiology with lab (1 semester), Organic Chemistry or Biochemistry with lab (1 semester)

Must have a 3.0 GPA or better in A+P, Micro, and Organic/Biochem and no more than two grades below C in any college level course. There may be at most one outstanding course in progress at the time of application.

D'YOUVILLE COLLEGE

Undergraduate
Admissions Office
D'Youville College

320 Porter Avenue
Buffalo, NY 14201
Phone: 716-829-7713
Email: paprogram@dyc.edu

Mission: The mission of the D'Youville College Physician Assistant Department is to prepare exemplary clinicians with the highest ethical standards, who will be leaders in the PA profession.

Accreditation: Continuing

Degree Offered: Combined BS/MS

Start Date: August annually

Program Length: 4.5 years

Class Capacity: 40 students

Tuition: $61,210 (pre-professional), $75,680 (professional) = $136,890

GPA Requirement: Overall GPA 3.0; also must rank in the top 25% of graduating high school class

Healthcare Experience: 80 hours required

PA Shadowing: Not required

Required Standardized Testing: Combined SAT score of at least 1100 (Math & Critical Reading sections) or a composite ACT score of 24 or higher

Letters of Recommendation: Three required; One should come from a healthcare provider or professional (i.e., a physician, RN, PA, etc.) who has observed the candidate in a healthcare setting (either volunteer or employed)

Seat Deposit: $150

CASPA Participant: Yes (for transfers only)

Supplemental Application: Additional PA application required if applying as a high school senior

Admissions: Rolling

Application Deadline: December 1

Prerequisite Coursework

Three years of math, one year of Chemistry and one year of Biology. Math and science subjects must have a minimum grade of at least 83 (B-).

No class statistics reported

PANCE Scores

5-year First Time Pass: 88%

Most Recent First Time Pass: 91%

Curriculum Structure

Pre-professional: 2 years

Didactic: 1 year

Clinical: 1.5 years

Rotations: 10 mandatory, 2 elective (ranging from 2-6 weeks)

Research Project: Required for graduation

Unique Program Features

Program: College freshmen who have not completed their first semester of freshman year may apply to transfer into the program. All other transfer students must apply through CASPA. See additional details on program's website.

PANCE Scores

5-year First Time Pass: 96%

Most Recent First Time Pass: 100%

Curriculum Structure

Didactic: 12 months

Clinical: 16 months (including a Research semester)

Rotations: 7 mandatory, 1 elective (each 6 weeks long)

Capstone Project: Required for graduation

Unique Program Features

Program: Option for a combined BS/MS program for students entering from high school.

HOFSTRA UNIVERSITY

Hofstra University
Email: paprogram@Hofstra.edu

113 Monroe Lecture Center
127 Hofstra University
Hempstead, NY 11549-1270
Phone: 516-463-4074

Mission: The mission of the Hofstra University Department of Physician Assistant Studies is to educate physician assistant students to provide health care with clinical excellence, compassion, and dedication to the community. The goals to meet this mission include: Train competent physician assistants qualified to practice evidence-based medicine in all clinical settings. Develop competence in oral and written communication skills. Provide the skills necessary for life-long learning. Express professionalism through respectful, compassionate and responsive interactions with patients, peers and supervisors. Encourage self-reflection in regard to the affective aspects of medical care. Impart pride of the physician assistant profession. Reinforce collaborative learning and working styles needed in order to participate in the team approach to medicine. Encourage the assumption of leadership roles within the profession and community. Inspire a desire among physician assistants toward service with underserved communities out of the mainstream of health care delivery.

Accreditation: Continuing

Degree Offered: Master (MSPAS)

Start Date: September annually

Program Length: 28 months

Class Capacity: 50 students

Tuition: $94,168

GPA Requirement: Overall GPA 3.2; Science GPA 3.2

Healthcare Experience: 50 hours required

PA Shadowing: Counts towards healthcare experience hours; no minimum number of hours needed

Required Standardized Testing: None

Letters of Recommendation: Two required; not from anyone specific

Seat Deposit: $1500

CASPA Participant: Yes
Supplemental Application: No

Admissions: Rolling
Application Deadline: October 1

Prerequisite Coursework

General Biology with lab (2 semesters), General Chemistry with lab (2 semesters), Human Physiology (1 semester), Human Anatomy (1 semester), Biochemistry or Organic Chemistry (1 semester), Microbiology (1 semester), Statistics (1 semester), Genetics or Cell Biology or other upper level Biology (1 semester)

LE MOYNE COLLEGE

Le Moyne College
Email: physassist@lemoyne.edu

1419 Salt Springs Road
Syracuse, NY 13214
Phone: 315-445-4745

Mission: The Le Moyne College Physician Assistant Program is dedicated to the education of students to become competent, caring, compassionate, and ethical providers of health care services with the supervision of a licensed physician. The program seeks to instill in each individual the desire to pursue a lifelong commitment to promote excellence in the delivery of patient care through continual self-assessment and advancement of one's medical skills and knowledge. The program prepares the student to work in a wide variety of settings under the supervision of licensed physicians, such as hospitals, private primary care facilities, nursing homes, and community centers.

Accreditation: Continuing

Degree Offered: Master (MS)

Start Date: August annually

Program Length: 24 months

Class Capacity: 75 students

Tuition: $77,162

CASPA Participant: Yes

Supplemental Application: No

Admissions: Not reported

Application Deadline: October 1

GPA Requirement:
Overall GPA 3.0;
Science GPA 3.0;
Prerequisite GPA 3.0

Healthcare Experience: 750 hours required

PA Shadowing: Counts towards healthcare experience hours; no specific number of hours required

Required Standardized Testing: None

Letters of Recommendation: Three required; One from an academic source and another from a professional in the health care field who can attest to your abilities

Seat Deposit: $750

No class statistics reported

PANCE Scores
5-year First Time Pass: 94%

Most Recent First Time Pass: 96%

Curriculum Structure
Didactic: 12 months
Clinical: 12 months
Rotations: 8 required (6 weeks each)
Masters Project: Required for graduation

Unique Program Features
Direct Entry: Direct entry option for exceptional college freshmen.

Curriculum: Le Moyne is one of only a handful of PA programs that presents medical humanities courses as an integral part of training.

Prerequisite Coursework

Biology with lab (2 semesters), Upper level Biology (4 courses); two of which must include lab, General Chemistry with lab (2 semesters), Organic Chemistry OR Biochemistry (1 semester), Statistics, Calculus or Physics (2 semesters), Social Science—Psychology courses, Sociology, Anthropology (2 semesters), English (1 semester). At least four advanced science courses must have been completed within the last five years.

PANCE Scores

5-year First Time Pass: 89%

Most Recent First Time Pass: 100%

Curriculum Structure

Didactic: 12 months

Clinical: 16 months

Rotations: 7 required, 1 medicine elective, 1 surgical elective, 1 clinical elective (all 5 weeks long)

Capstone Project: Required for graduation

Unique Program Features

Not reported

LONG ISLAND UNIVERSITY

Long Island University
Email:
bkln-PAStudies@liu.edu

1 University Plaza
Brooklyn, NY 11201
Phone: 718-488-1505

Mission: The Division of Physician Assistant Studies supports the University's mission by educating men and women of all ethnic and socioeconomic backgrounds in the art and science of medicine so that they may become highly competent and compassionate physician assistants. The program will advance medical knowledge and contribute to the PA profession through community service and scholarship.

Accreditation: Continuing

Degree Offered: Master (MSPAS)

Start Date: August annually

Program Length: 28 months

Class Capacity: 42 students

Tuition: $97,180

GPA Requirement: Overall GPA 3.0; Science GPA 3.0; Prerequisite GPA 3.0

Healthcare Experience: 500 hours required

PA Shadowing: Counts towards healthcare experience hours; no specific number of hours required

Required Standardized Testing: GRE

Letters of Recommendation: Three required; not from anyone specific

Seat Deposit: $500

CASPA Participant: Yes

Supplemental Application: No

Admissions: Not reported

Application Deadline: January 15

Prerequisite Coursework

General Biology with lab (2 semesters), General Chemistry with lab (2 semesters), Human Anatomy with lab (1 semester), Human Physiology with lab (1 semester), Microbiology (1 semester), Statistics (1 semester)

MERCY COLLEGE

Mercy College
Email:
PAProgram@mercy.edu

1200 Waters Place
Bronx, NY 10461
Phone: 914-674-7635

Mission: The mission of the Mercy College Graduate Program in Physician Assistant Studies is to educate physician assistants to provide quality, cost-effective, accessible health care, especially to underserved patients in the Tri-state area.

Accreditation:
Continuing

Degree Offered:
Master (MSPAS)

Start Date:
June annually

Program Length:
27 months

Class Capacity:
65 students

Tuition: $88,000

GPA Requirement:
Overall GPA 3.0;
Science GPA 3.2

Healthcare Experience:
500 hours required; 250 hours must be completed in a primary care setting such as family medicine, outpatient internal medicine, pediatrics, or OB/GYN

PA Shadowing: Not required

Required Standardized Testing: Not required

Letters of Recommendation: Three required; One must be from a PA, MD, or work supervisor

Seat Deposit: $800

CASPA Participant: Yes

Supplemental Application: Yes

Admissions: Not reported

Application Deadline:
November 1

Prerequisite Coursework

Biology with lab (2 semesters), Microbiology with lab (1 semester), Human Physiology (1 semester), Upper level Biology (1 semester), Chemistry with lab (2 semesters), Biochemistry (1 semester), Statistics (1 semester)

No more than 75 credits can be from a two-year college. Biochemistry, Microbiology, and Human Physiology must have been taken within 5 years and 2 of the 3 courses must be completed at a 4-year institution. Upper level Biology must be taken at a 4-year institution.

No class statistics reported

PANCE Scores
5-year First Time Pass: 87%

Most Recent First Time Pass: 90%

Curriculum Structure
Didactic: 12 months
Clinical: 15 months
Rotations: 7 required, 1 primary care elective, 1 elective (six are 6 weeks long, three are 4 weeks long)
Capstone Project: Required for graduation

Unique Program Features

Foreign Language: Medical Spanish is required as part of the curriculum.

Community Service: The program participates in international medical missions and students and faculty operate a mobile health vehicle that provides health screenings and education to members of the community twice a month.

Class of 2018
Male: 20%
Female: 80%
Minority: Not reported
GPA: 3.8
Science GPA: 3.7
GRE: Not required
Faculty to Student Ratio: Not reported
Average Healthcare Experience: Not reported

PANCE Scores
5-year First Time Pass: 92%

Most Recent First Time Pass: 92%

Curriculum Structure
Didactic: 18 months
Clinical: 12 months
Rotations: 8 mandatory (three are 8 weeks long, five are 4 weeks long), 1 elective (4 weeks long)
Research Project: Required for graduation

CASPA Participant: Yes

Supplemental Application: No

New York Institute of Technology
Email: pa@nyit.edu

PA Department, Riland Room 352
Northern Boulevard, PO Box 8000
Old Westbury, NY 11568-8000
Phone: 516-686-3881

Mission: The mission of the Physician Assistant Program is based on the fundamental principles of New York Institute of Technology, the Physician Assistant Profession and the belief that access for all persons to quality health care is a right. The mission includes educating physician assistant students to provide high quality healthcare services to all segments of the population throughout the country; become culturally sensitive and caring; integrate academic knowledge with practice. The NYIT Physician Assistant Program seeks and encourages diversity in the recruitment of minorities within its faculty, staff, and student body, provides an interdisciplinary educational experience which includes the holistic approach to patients, enhances the students' educational experience through the integration of the technological resources of New York Institute of Technology

Accreditation: Continuing

Degree Offered: Master (MSPAS)

Start Date: September annually

Program Length: 30 months

Class Capacity: 56 students

Tuition: $113,190

Admissions: Not rolling

Application Deadline: October 1

GPA Requirement: Overall GPA 3.0

Healthcare Experience: 100 hours required

PA Shadowing: Counts towards healthcare experience hours; no minimum number of hours needed

Required Standardized Testing: Not required

Letters of Recommendation: Three required; One from a PA, MD, or DO, one professional or faculty letter, and one other professional or faculty letter

Seat Deposit: $1500

Prerequisite Coursework

Biology (2 semesters; no lab requirement), Human Anatomy and Physiology (2 semesters), Chemistry with lab (2 semesters), Psychology (1 semester) Math (2 semesters). All prerequisites must be completed with a grade of "B-" or better.

Unique Program Features

Pre-PA Program: Option for 6-year combined BS/MS program for students entering from high school.

Didactics: Didactic coursework is spread out over two years instead of one with a summer break after completion of year 1.

Facilities: The department has a dedicated classroom/laboratory with audio-visual equipment, X-Ray Viewing Box, two electrocardiograph machines, and various human patient simulator models used for skills training. A state-of-the-art standardized patient laboratory has been developed for use by medical and physician assistant students to enhance skill acquisition. A cadaver lab provides a valuable hands-on approach to learning anatomy.

PACE UNIVERSITY

Pace University Department of Physician Assistant Studies

College of Health Professions
163 William Street, 5th floor
New York, NY 10038
Phone: 212-618-6052
Email: paprogram_admissions@pace.edu

Mission: The mission of the Pace University-Lenox Hill Hospital Physician Assistant Program is to conduct a quality education program that produces superior physician assistants who possess the requisite skills, knowledge, attitude and understanding to function in diverse communities, populations, and settings, and to treat all patients with dignity, respect and compassion.

Accreditation:
Continuing

Degree Offered:
Master (MSPAS)

Start Date:
July annually

Program Length:
26 months

Class Capacity:
80 students

Tuition: $94,965

GPA Requirement: Overall GPA 3.0; Science GPA 3.0;

Healthcare Experience:
200 hours

PA Shadowing: Not required

Required Standardized Testing: None

Letters of Recommendation:
Three required; at least one should be from a healthcare professional

Seat Deposit: $1,500

CASPA Participant: Yes

Supplemental Application: No

Admissions: Not reported

Application Deadline:
August 1

Class of 2017
Male: 22%
Female: 78%
Minority: Not reported
GPA: 3.58
Science GPA: 3.54
GRE: Not required
Faculty to Student Ratio: Not reported
Average Healthcare Experience: 1,847 hours

PANCE Scores
5-year First Time Pass: 98%

Most Recent First Time Pass: 99%

Curriculum Structure
Didactic: 14 months
Clinical: 12 months
Rotations: 8 mandatory, 1 elective (all 5 weeks long)
Research Method/ Master Project: Required for graduation

Prerequisite Coursework

Anatomy with lab (1 semester), Physiology (1 semester), General Biology with lab (2 semesters), General Chemistry with lab (2 semesters), Organic Chemistry or Biochemistry with lab (1 semester), Precalculus or Statistics (1 semester), Microbiology (1 semester).There can be no more than one grade that is less than a "B-" in a required prerequisite course. All prerequisites must be completed at the time of application e-submission to CASPA.

Unique Program Features

Community Service: The Pace PA program is involved in a number of different volunteer projects throughout the year and raises funds for charitable organizations like the Susan G. Komen foundation and Leukemia and Lymphoma society.

Rotations: The program boasts access to rotation sites in all five NYC boroughs as well as Connecticut and New Jersey. They also offer international rotation opportunities.

No class statistics

PANCE Scores

5-year First Time Pass: 95%

Most Recent First Time Pass: 89%

Curriculum Structure

Pre-professional: 2 years of undergraduate coursework

Didactic: 18 months

Clinical: 12 months

Rotations: 9 required, 1 elective

Capstone Project: Required for graduation

Unique Program Features

Dual Degree: RIT is transitioning to a dual BS/MS program. Transfer students are accepted.

ROCHESTER INSTITUTE OF TECHNOLOGY

Rochester Institute of Technology
Office of Admissions - Bausch & Lomb Center

60 Lomb Memorial Drive
Rochester, NY 14623
Phone: 585-475-5151
Email: llwscl@rit.edu

Mission: The Rochester Institute of Technology Physician Assistant Program, built on a foundation of liberal arts and sciences, will prepare students to provide compassionate, high quality patient and health care services. Fundamental to the Program is a commitment to develop within students and faculty the values and skills necessary for the pursuit of life-long learning and dedication to community service.

Accreditation: Continuing

Degree Offered: BS/MS

Start Date: September annually

Program Length: 30 months

Class Capacity: 36 students

Tuition: $193,666 for the total 5 year program

GPA Requirement: Overall GPA 3.0; Science GPA 3.0;

Healthcare Experience: Preferred/Recommended

PA Shadowing: Not required

Required Standardized Testing: None

Letters of Recommendation: Two required; not from anyone specific

Seat Deposit: $300

CASPA Participant: No

Supplemental Application: Yes

Admissions: Not reported; early decision available

Application Deadline: December 1

Prerequisite Coursework

Not specifically mentioned; see program website for additional information

STONY BROOK

Stony Brook
University
School of Technology
and Management

Health Science, Level 2 Room 428
Stony Brook, NY 11794-8202
Phone: 631-444-3190
Email: paprogram@stonybrook.edu

Mission: The mission of the Stony Brook University Physician Assistant Program is to provide high quality graduate-level medical education in an interprofessional environment that fosters critical thinking and life-long learning. We seek to develop in our students the knowledge, attitudes, and skills necessary to be outstanding, compassionate health care providers. We promote professionalism, leadership, service and an appreciation of ethical values and diversity. Physician assistant education at Stony Brook emphasizes comprehensive patient-centered medical care across the lifespan and our curriculum focuses on the principles of evidence-based practice and the importance of scholarly activity.

PANCE Scores

5-year First Time Pass: 97%

Most Recent First Time Pass: 98%

Curriculum Structure

Didactic: 12 months

Clinical: 12 months

Rotations: 9 mandatory (seven are 5 weeks long, two are 4 weeks long), 1 elective (4 weeks long)

Masters Project: Required for graduation

Unique Program Features

Applying: Applicants should have a strong leadership and community service background to be competitive.

Community Service: Students and faculty are involved in a number of international medical mission trips.

Accreditation: Continuing

Degree Offered: Master (MS)

Start Date: June annually

Program Length: 24 months

Class Capacity: 44 students

Tuition: $35,368 (in-state); $79,220 (out-of-state)

GPA Requirement: Overall GPA 3.0; Science GPA 3.0

Healthcare Experience: 1,000 hours required

PA Shadowing: Counts towards healthcare experience hours; only 200 hours of shadowing can be put toward the 1000 hour requirement for healthcare experience

Required Standardized Testing: Not required

Letters of Recommendation: Three required; One academic letter, one health care letter, and one from a PA

Seat Deposit: None

CASPA Participant: Yes

Supplemental Application: Yes

Admissions: Rolling

Application Deadline: October 1

Prerequisite Coursework

General Biology (2 semesters), Anatomy (1 semester), Physiology (1 semester), General Chemistry (2 semesters), Biochemistry (1 semester), Organic Chemistry (1 semester), Microbiology (1 semester), Genetics (1 semester), Statistics or Biostatistics (1 semester), Arts/Humanities such as philosophy, literature, art, music, religion (2 semesters), Social/Behavioral Science such as psychology, sociology, history, economics, anthropology (3 semesters or 9 credit hours), English Composition (1 semester). Only one of the natural science courses may be outstanding at the time of application.

PANCE Scores

5-year First Time Pass: 90%

Most Recent First Time Pass: 92%

Curriculum Structure

Didactic: 15 months

Clinical: 12 months

Rotations: 8 mandatory, 1 medicine elective, 1 surgery elective (six are 6 weeks, four are 3 weeks)

Capstone Project: None

Unique Program Features

None reported

SUNY DOWNSTATE MEDICAL CENTER

SUNY Downstate Medical Center
Email: PA.CHRP@downstate.edu

450 Clarkson Avenue
Box 1222
Brooklyn, NY 11203
Phone: 718-270-2324/2325

Mission: The mission of the SUNY Downstate Physician Assistant Program is to educate health care professionals in the delivery of excellent health care service.

Accreditation: Continuing

Degree Offered: Bachelor (BS)

Start Date: June annually, beginning in the Junior Year

Program Length: 27 months

Class Capacity: 35 students

Tuition: Varies by track and in-state vs. out-of-state; see program website for more information

GPA Requirement: Overall GPA 3.0

Healthcare Experience: 225 hours required

PA Shadowing: Recommended but no specific number of hours required

Volunteer Experience: Required (150 hours)

Required Standardized Testing: Not required

Letters of Recommendation: Two required; One should be from a clinician (PA, MD, NP, etc.)

Seat Deposit: $150

CASPA Participant: No

Supplemental Application: No

Admissions: Early applications are encouraged

Application Deadline: November 30

Prerequisite Coursework

Anatomy and Physiology I and II with lab (2 semesters), General Biology I and II with lab (2 semesters), General Chemistry I and II with lab (2 semesters), Microbiology with lab (1 semester), Math (1 semester), General Psychology (1 semester), Abnormal Psychology OR Life Span Psychology (1 semester), English (2 semesters), Humanities/Social Science (2 semesters), Upper level science (1 semester). All prerequisite courses should have been completed within 8 years of the matriculation date.

SUNY UPSTATE

SUNY Upstate Medical Center
Email: admissfa@upstate.edu

750 E. Adams Street
Syracuse, NY 13210
Phone: 315-464-6561

Mission: The mission of the Physician Assistant Program is to educate highly qualified physician assistants with patient centered values who practice medicine confidently and ethically by demonstrating academic excellence and clinical competence. Our emphasis is on serving the medically underserved populations in Upstate New York.

Accreditation: Continuing

Degree Offered: Master (MSPAS)

Start Date: June annually

Program Length: 27 months

Class Capacity: 35 students

Tuition: $32,150 in-state; $62,425 out-of-state

GPA Requirement: Overall GPA 3.0

Healthcare Experience: 1,000 hours required

PA Shadowing: Strongly recommended but no specific number of hours required

Required Standardized Testing: GRE

Letters of Recommendation: Three required; One academic letter, one professional letter, and one letter from a PA

Seat Deposit: $150

CASPA Participant: Yes

Supplemental Application: Yes

Admissions: Rolling

Application Deadline: December 1

PANCE Scores

5-year First Time Pass: 91%

Most Recent First Time Pass: 94%

Curriculum Structure

Didactic: 15 months

Clinical: 12 months

Rotations: 9 mandatory, 2 electives (all 4 weeks long)

Capstone Project: Required for graduation

Unique Program Features

None reported

Prerequisite Coursework

Anatomy and Physiology I and II with lab (2 semesters), General Biology I and II with lab (2 semesters), General Chemistry I and II with lab (2 semesters), Organic Chemistry OR Biochemistry with lab (1 semester), Microbiology with lab (1 semester), Genetics (1 semester), Statistics (1 semester), English (2 semesters, including composition), Medical Terminology, Behavioral/Social Science (2 semesters), One biology and one chemistry course need to be taken within 5 years of matriculation into the PA program.

Class of 2014
GPA: 3.4

PANCE Scores

5-year First Time Pass: 97%

Most Recent First Time Pass: 98% (Bay Shore); 100% (Winthrop)

Curriculum Structure

Didactic: 12 months

Clinical: 12 months

Rotations: 7 mandatory, 2 elective (all 5 weeks long)

Research Project: Required for graduation

Unique Program Features

None reported

TOURO COLLEGE—BAY SHORE AND WINTHROP EXTENSION CENTER

Touro College School of Health Sciences
Physician Assistant Program/Office of Admissions
1700 Union Boulevard
Bay Shore, NY 11706

Touro College Winthrop University Hospital Extension Center
288 Old Country Road
Mineola, NY 11501
Phone: 631-665-1600
Email: enrollhealth@touro.edu

Mission: : The mission of the Touro College Physician Assistant Programs is to educate capable students to meet the challenges of providing health care services under the supervision of a licensed physician. The programs also strive to excel in the education and training of physician assistants who will serve the health care needs of the community with competence, compassion, and dedication. The program curriculum is designed to educate its graduates to function as traditionally-trained primary care providers who are able to provide care to patients in any number of specialties in hospital-based and private office settings, and to prepare graduates with the requisite medical knowledge to pass the national certifying examination.

Accreditation: Continuing

Degree Offered: Bachelor (BS) and Master (MSPAS)

Start Date: August annually (Bay Shore); January annually (Winthrop)

Program Length: 24 months

Class Capacity: 65 students (Bay Shore); 32 students (Winthrop)

Tuition: $86,440

GPA Requirement: Overall GPA 3.0; Science GPA 3.0

Healthcare Experience: 200 hours required

PA Shadowing: Required (20 hours)

Required Standardized Testing: Not required

Letters of Recommendation: Three required; One must be from a PA

Seat Deposit: $1500

CASPA Participant: Yes

Supplemental Application: Yes

Admissions: Not reported

Application Deadline: March 1 (Bay Shore); November 1 (Winthrop)

Prerequisite Coursework

General Biology I and II with lab (2 semesters), General Chemistry I and II with lab (2 semesters), Organic Chemistry OR Biochemistry (1 semester), Anatomy and Physiology I and II (2 semesters), Behavioral Science (2 semesters), English (2 semesters), Humanities (2 semesters), Math—pre-calculus or above (1 semester), Statistics (1 semester)

TOURO COLLEGE——MANHATTAN

Physician Assistant Program/Office of Admissions
Touro College School of Health Sciences

1700 Union Boulevard
Bay Shore, NY 11706
Phone: 646-795-4510
Email: enrollhealth@touro.edu

PANCE Scores

5-year First Time Pass: 88%

Most Recent First Time Pass: 100%

Mission: The mission of the Touro College Physician Assistant Programs is to educate capable students to meet the challenges of providing health care services under the supervision of a licensed physician. The programs also strive to excel in the education and training of physician assistants who will serve the health care needs of the community with competence, compassion, and dedication.

Curriculum Structure

Didactic: 16 months (evening classes and Sundays)

Clinical: 16 months

Rotations: 8 mandatory, 2 elective (all 5 weeks long)

Capstone Project: Required for graduation

Accreditation: Continuing

Degree Offered: Bachelor (BS) and Master (MSPAS)

Start Date: August annually

Program Length: 32 months (non-traditional)

Class Capacity: 50 students

Tuition: $89,124

GPA Requirement: Overall GPA 3.0; Science GPA 3.0

Healthcare Experience: 200 hours required

PA Shadowing: Required (20 hours)

Required Standardized Testing: Not required

Letters of Recommendation: Three required; One must be from a PA

Seat Deposit: $1,500

Unique Program Features

Timing: This program accommodates individuals who wish to embark on a career as a PA but may have other life circumstances that prevent them from being to participate in the traditional didactic curriculum.

CASPA Participant: Yes

Supplemental Application: Yes

Admissions: Not reported

Application Deadline: January 15; early decision November 1

Prerequisite Coursework

General Biology I and II with lab (2 semesters), General Chemistry I and II with lab (2 semesters), Organic Chemistry OR Biochemistry (1 semester), Anatomy and Physiology I and II (2 semesters), Behavioral Science (2 semesters), English (2 semesters), Humanities (2 semesters)

Math—pre-calculus or above (1 semester), Statistics (1 semester)

PANCE Scores

5-year First Time Pass: 93%

Most Recent First Time Pass: 96%

Curriculum Structure

Pre-professional: 2 years

Didactic: 15 months

Clinical: 21 months

Rotations: 7 mandatory

Thesis Project: Required for graduation

Unique Program Features

Direct Entry: Direct entry track for college freshmen for combined BS/MS degree available.

Scholarship: Wagner College offers an unlimited number of renewable $4,000 per year ($2,000 per semester) scholarships for members of Phi Theta Kappa. Part-time students and students with previous bachelor's degrees are not eligible. Proof of Phi Theta Kappa membership is required.

WAGNER COLLEGE

Wagner College

One Campus Road
Staten Island, NY 10301
Phone: 718-420-4151

Mission: To prepare professional academic clinicians committed to providing quality health care to all individuals.

Accreditation: Continuing

Degree Offered: Certificate, Master (MS)

Start Date: June annually

Program Length: 36 months

Class Capacity: 40 students

Tuition: $91,888

GPA Requirement: Overall GPA 3.2; Science GPA 3.0; Prerequisite GPA 3.0

Healthcare Experience: Not reported

PA Shadowing: Not reported

Volunteer Experience: 100 hours required

Required Standardized Testing: None

Letters of Recommendation: Three required; Preferably from faculty

Seat Deposit: Not reported

CASPA Participant: No

Supplemental Application: No

Admissions: Not reported

Application Deadline: December 1

Prerequisite Coursework

Human Anatomy and Physiology I and II (2 semesters), General Chemistry I and II (2 semesters), Organic Chemistry (1 semester), Microbiology (1 semester)

Pathology (1 semester), Philosophy/Medical Ethics (1 semester), Introduction to Psychology (1 semester), Biostatistics and Experimental Design OR Statistics (1 semester)

NORTH CAROLINA

CAMPBELL UNIVERSITY

Campbell University
College of Pharmacy
& Health Sciences
Attention: PA Program

PO Box 1090
Buies Creek, NC 27506
Phone: 910-893-1210
Email: paga@campbell.edu

Mission: Campbell University's Physician Assistant (PA) program provides graduate professional clinical education in a Christian environment. Solid principles of science and research are integrated using the highest ethical and professional standards, while developing a vision to the future of the PA profession and its role in the healthcare delivery system. The PA program promotes patient centered, evidence-based medicine preparing students to be compassionate, competent healthcare providers with an emphasis on primary care, health promotion and disease prevention.

Accreditation:
Continued
Degree Offered:
Master (MPAP)
Start Date:
August annually
Program Length:
24 months
Class Capacity: 44
students
Tuition: $70,800

CASPA Participant:
Yes
Supplemental Application: Yes
Admissions: Rolling
Application Deadline:
November 1

GPA Requirement:
Overall GPA 3.2;
Science GPA 3.2;
Prerequisite GPA 3.2
Healthcare Experience: 1,000 hours required
PA Shadowing: 20 hours recommended, not required
Required Standardized Testing: GRE (preference for those with scores > 50th percentile)
Letters of Recommendation:
Three required; preference is given to applicants with two out of three letters from physicians, PAs or clinical supervisors, and others familiar with your clinical experience
Seat Deposit: $1500

Class of 2017
Male: not reported
Female: not reported
Minority:
not reported
GPA: 3.45
Science GPA:
not reported
GREVerbal: 162
GRE Quantitative:
167
GRE Writing: 4.1
Faculty to Student Ratio: not reported
Average Healthcare Experience:
5,930 hours

PANCE Scores
5-year First Time Pass:
92% (based on two years of data)
Most Recent First Time Pass: 95%

Curriculum Structure
Didactic: 12 months
Clinical: 12 months
Rotations:
8 mandatory, 2 elective; 4 weeks each
Evidence-Based Medicine Paper:
required for graduation

Prerequisite Coursework

General Biology (1 semester), Human Anatomy and Physiology with lab (2 semesters), Microbiology with lab (1 semester), General Chemistry with lab (1 semester), Organic Chemistry or Biochemistry (1 semester), Statistics or Biostatistics (1 semester), Psychology (1 semester). All prerequisites must be completed no later than 12/31 of the year prior to matriculation.

Unique Program Features

Dual Degree Program:
Campbell University offers the only PA/MS in Public Health dual degree program in North Carolina, providing PA students with a solid foundation in health care research and outcomes evaluation.

Facilities: The Hall of Medical Sciences is a 96,500 square foot facility that contains a simulation center for standardized patients, a physical assessment lab, 12 OSCE rooms, and an anatomy lab. It includes student group rooms, a resource library, a small café, and sophisticated technical equipment for hands-on, real-life application.

Community Service: The Wallace Student Society completes community service project with a focus on prevention and health promotion in rural communities through patient education and charity fundraising.

Class of 2017

Male: not reported
Female: not reported
Minority: not reported
GPA: 3.4-3.8 (interquartile range)
Science GPA: 3.3-3.8 (interquartile range)
GRE Verbal: 155-161 (interquartile range)
GRE Quantitative: 153-158 (interquartile range)
GRE Writing: 4.0-4.5 (interquartile range)
Faculty to Student Ratio: not reported
Average Healthcare Experience: 16-43 months

PANCE Scores

5-year First Time Pass: 96%
Most Recent First Time Pass: 99%

Curriculum Structure

Didactic: 12 months
Clinical: 12 months
Rotations: 8 mandatory, 2 elective; 4-8 weeks each

DUKE UNIVERSITY MEDICAL CENTER

Duke University
Email: paadmission@mc.duke.edu

Physician Assistant Program, Box 10780 DUMC
Durham, NC 27710
Phone: 919-681-3161

Mission: The Duke Physician Assistant Program's mission is to educate caring, competent primary care physician assistants who practice evidence-based medicine, are leaders in the profession, dedicated to their communities, culturally sensitive, and devoted to positive transformation of the health care system.

Accreditation: Continued
Degree Offered: Master (MHS)
Start Date: August annually
Program Length: 24 months
Class Capacity: 90 students
Tuition: $77,714

GPA Requirement: None
Healthcare Experience: 1,000 hours required
PA Shadowing: Not required
Required Standardized Testing: GRE
Letters of Recommendation: Three required; one from a medical professional or supervisor and two letters of the applicant's choice
Seat Deposit: $1,125

CASPA Participant: Yes
Supplemental Application: Yes

Admissions: Rolling
Application Deadline: October 1

Prerequisite Coursework

Anatomy (3 credits), Physiology (3 credits), Microbiology (3 credits), Other Biology (6 credits), Chemistry with lab (8 credits), Statistics (2 credits). All courses must be completed by the end of the fall semester prior to matriculation.

Unique Program Features

History: The PA profession originated at Duke in the mid-1960s with Dr. Eugene Stead and thus Duke is the oldest PA program in the nation.
Community Service: Students in the Duke PA Program have a long tradition of taking time out of their busy academic schedules to participate in community service and fundraising. Specific opportunities are available to view on their website and have included involvement in diaper drives, food drives, trash collection, Habitat for Humanity, and others.
Research: Duke has established a research section to advance scholarship on the PA profession.
Student Blog: A first and second year student blog is maintained to allow applicants to understand a typical day in the life of a PA student at Duke and explore their experiences.

EAST CAROLINA UNIVERSITY

East Carolina University
Email:
PAAdmissions@ecu.edu

600 Moye Boulevard
Mail Stop 668
Greenville, NC 27834
Phone: 252-744-1100

Mission: The mission of the Physician Assistant Studies program is to provide educational experiences which prepare physician assistant graduates to enhance the access to primary medical care for the citizens of rural and medically underserved eastern North Carolina and beyond in an educational community where faculty, staff, clinical instructors, students, and other health care providers work together in an atmosphere of mutual respect, cooperation, compassion and commitment.

Accreditation:
Continued

Degree Offered:
Master (MSPA)

Start Date:
August annually

Program Length:
27 months

Class Capacity:
35 students

Tuition:
In-state: $33,970;
Out-of-state: $80,310
(tuition + fees)

GPA Requirement:
Overall GPA 3.0

Healthcare Experience:
1,000 hours required

PA Shadowing: 250 hours preferred, not required

Required Standardized Testing: GRE

Letters of Recommendation: Three required; prefer that your references come from medical professionals, supervisors, and professors

Seat Deposit: None

CASPA Participant: Yes

Supplemental Application: No

Admissions: Rolling

Application Deadline:
September 1

Unique Program Features

Admissions Preference: Applicants must be residents of North Carolina, South Carolina, Virginia, Tennessee, or Georgia with preference given to those from North Carolina. 35-50% of accepted students are typically from rural communities.

Student Blog: A student blog is maintained where students periodically comment about their experiences at the University which is available to view for prospective applicants on the website.

Rotation Sites: Most of the rotation sites are found in healthcare provider shortage areas, in line with the mission of the program to help relieve this shortage in North Carolina.

Class of 2016
Male: not reported
Female: not reported
Minority:
not reported
GPA: 3.78
Science GPA: 3.76
GRECombined: 312
GRE Writing: 4.24
Faculty to Student Ratio: not reported
Average Healthcare Experience:
not reported

PANCE Scores
5-year First Time Pass:
97%
Most Recent First Time Pass: 100%

Curriculum Structure
Didactic: 15months
Clinical: 12 months
Rotations:
8 mandatory;
4-8 weeks each

Prerequisite Coursework
Human Anatomy and Physiology I and II with lab (8 credits), Genetics (3 credits), General Chemistry or higher with lab (8 credits), Microbiology (3 credits), Psychology (3 credits), Statistics (3 credits), Medical Terminology (1 credit). They prefer all courses be completed in the last 7 years and applicants may have one pending prerequisite course as long as it is completed by December 31.

Class of 2018

Male: 21%
Female: 79%
Minority: not reported
GPA: 3.65
Science GPA: 3.62
GREVerbal: 155
GRE Quantitative: 155
GRE Writing: 4.0
Faculty to Student Ratio: not reported
Average Healthcare Experience: 2,341

PANCE Scores

5-year First Time Pass: N/A (only one year of data reported)

Most Recent First Time Pass: 100%

Curriculum Structure

Didactic: 12months
Clinical: 15 months
Rotations: 7 mandatory, 2 electives; 6 weeks each
Master's Project: Required for graduation

ELON UNIVERSITY

Elon University
Email:
gradadm@elon.edu

2750 Campus Box
Elon, NC 27244
Phone: 336-278-7600

Mission: The Elon University Department of Physician Assistant Studies embraces the overall mission of the University and seeks to fulfill the Departmental vision of "Learning. Caring. Serving. Leading."

Accreditation: Provisional

Degree Offered: Master (MSPA)

Start Date: January annually

Program Length: 27 months

Class Capacity: 38 students

Tuition: In-state: $80,370

GPA Requirement: Overall GPA 3.2; Science GPA 3.0

Healthcare Experience: 250 hours required

PA Shadowing: 20 hours required

Required Standardized Testing: GRE

Letters of Recommendation: Three required; including one from a Physician Assistant or other healthcare provider; and two others.

Seat Deposit: $1,000

CASPA Participant: Yes
Supplemental Application: No

Admissions: Rolling
Application Deadline: November 1

Unique Program Features

Facilities: The physician assistant studies program's dedicated teaching space includes two classrooms, a clinical skills laboratory, five simulated exam rooms, a cardiopulmonary auscultation lab, wet dissection/clinical procedure lab and six small group study rooms.

Global Learning Opportunity: Elon University School of Health Sciences has a program to develop global clinicians and informed leaders through clinical or service-learning experience that takes place in a culturally unique clinical setting with cultural immersion.

Prerequisite Coursework

Anatomy and Physiology (7 credits), General Chemistry with lab (4 credits), Additional Chemistry with lab (4 credits), Upper Level Science (6 credits), Upper Level Human Conditions Courses (6 credits). Science courses should have been completed in the last 10 years and five of six science courses should be completed at the time of application.

GARDNER WEBB UNIVERSITY

Gardner Webb University
Email: paprogram @gardner-webb.edu

110 S. Main Street
Boiling Springs, NC 28017
Phone: 704-406-2369

Mission: Develop knowledgeable and caring Physician Assistants who practice competent patient-centered primary care in diverse environments.

Accreditation: Provisional

Degree Offered: Master (MPAS)

Start Date: January annually

Program Length: 28 months

Class Capacity: 36 students

Tuition: $78,308

GPA Requirement: Overall GPA 3.0; Prerequisite GPA 2.7

Healthcare Experience: Preferred, not required.

PA Shadowing: Not required

Required Standardized Testing: GRE

Letters of Recommendation: Three required; health care provider preferable for at least one reference

Seat Deposit: $1,500

CASPA Participant: Yes

Supplemental Application: No

Admissions: Rolling

Application Deadline: October 1

Prerequisite Coursework

Human Anatomy and Physiology I and II with lab (2 semesters), General Biology with lab (1 semester), Other Biology with lab (1 semester), Microbiology with lab (1 semester), General Chemistry with lab (1 semester), Other Chemistry with lab (1 semester), Organic Chemistry with lab (1 semester), Statistics (1 course), Psychology (1 course), Medical Terminology (1 course). Two courses may be in progress at the time of application but must be completed the summer semester prior to matriculation.

Unique Program Features

Underserved Focus: All students will complete a 3 week clinical rotation with an underserved population, in line with the programs service values. The program is also developing international mission opportunities for students.

PANCE Scores

5-year First Time Pass: N/A

Most Recent First Time Pass: N/A (no classes have graduated yet)

Curriculum Structure

Didactic: 15 months

Clinical: 12 months

Rotations: 7 mandatory, 2 electives; 5 weeks each

Master's Project: Required for graduation

Prerequisite Coursework

Human or Vertebrate Anatomy with lab (4 credits), Human or Vertebrate Physiology (3 credits), Biological Science with lab (8 credits), Upper Level Human Biological Science (3 credits), Microbiology (3 credits), General/Inorganic Chemistry with lab (4 credits), Additional Chemistry with lab (4 credits), Statistics (3 credits), Psychology (3 credits), Humanities and Social Sciences (9 credits, at least one upper level course). Medical Terminology is required but can be completed post-acceptance. Only one prerequisite course can be in progress during the Fall semester of the year you apply and science courses must have been taken in the last 10 years.

HIGH POINT UNIVERSITY

High Point University
Email: PAprogram@highpoint.edu

Office of Graduate Admissions Drawer 26
833 Montlieu Avenue
High Point, NC 27282
Phone: 336-841-9504

Mission: : The mission of the High Point University Physician Assistant Studies program is to deliver a student-centered, experiential curriculum grounded in high academic and ethical standards. The program strives to develop compassionate physician assistants who are self-directed lifelong learners prepared to provide evidence-based, patient-centered care as members of an inter-professional health care team.

Accreditation: Provisional

Degree Offered: Master (MPAS)

Start Date: June annually

Program Length: 27 months

Class Capacity: 20 students

Tuition: $80,068

GPA Requirement: Overall GPA 3.2; Science GPA 3.2

Healthcare Experience: 200 hours required

PA Shadowing: 15 hours required

Required Standardized Testing: GRE

Letters of Recommendation: Three required; recommended one from professor and one from a supervisor.

Seat Deposit: $1,000

CASPA Participant: Yes

Supplemental Application: No

Admissions: Rolling

Application Deadline: October 1

Unique Program Features

Students First: The faculty is committed to maximizing the students educational experience through innovative and stimulating learning experiences, mentoring relationships with students, small student to faculty ratios, and feedback and support for professional development.

Experiential Learning: The program provides opportunities for medical simulation, standardized patients, task trainers, problem-based learning, case-based learning, team-based learning and other emerging technologies.

Staying Ahead of the Curve: The program is committed to preparing healthcare professionals for the world as it is going to be in the future through maximizing the use of health information technology.

LENOIR-RHYNE UNIVERSITY

Lenoir-Rhyne University Physician Assistant Program

625 7th Avenue NE
Hickory, NC 28601
Phone: 828-328-7129
Email: kelly.powell@lr.edu

Mission: : The Mission of the Master of Science in Physician Assistant Studies Program is to educate highly qualified physician assistants from diverse faith, geographic, socioeconomic and cultural backgrounds; preparing them to become competent and compassionate health care professionals, providing quality healthcare to diverse populations in medically underserved areas locally, nationally and internationally.

Accreditation: Provisional

Degree Offered: Master (MSPAS)

Start Date: January annually

Program Length: 27 months

Class Capacity: 48 students

Tuition: $77,000

CASPA Participant: Yes

Supplemental Application: No

Admissions: Rolling

Application Deadline: October 1

GPA Requirement: Overall GPA 3.0; Science GPA 3.0; Prerequisite GPA 3.0

Healthcare Experience: Recommended, not required

PA Shadowing: Encouraged, not required

Required Standardized Testing: GRE (>301 preferred; applicants with graduate degree are exempt)

Letters of Recommendation: Three required; one from a Medical provider (MD, DO, PA, and NP), one from a Professor and one from an employer or coach

Seat Deposit: $1,000

No class statistics reported

PANCE Scores

5-year First Time Pass: N/A

Most Recent First Time Pass: N/A (no classes have graduated yet)

Curriculum Structure

Didactic: 15 months

Clinical: 12 months

Rotations: 7 mandatory, 1 electives; 6 weeks each

Capstone Project: Required for graduation

Unique Program Features

Not specified

Prerequisite Coursework

Biology I and II with Lab, Microbiology with lab, Chemistry I and II with lab, Organic Chemistry I and II with lab, Biochemistry with lab, Anatomy and Physiology I and II with lab, Psychology, Sociology or Social Science, Two upper-level math courses (one must be statistics), Medical Terminology, Genetics, Physics. Students can apply with two pending prerequisites.

Class of 2017

Male: not reported

Female: not reported

Minority: not reported

GPA: 3.57

Prerequisite GPA: 3.65

GRECombined: 306

GRE Writing: not reported

Faculty to Student Ratio: not reported

Average Healthcare Experience: 2,500 hours

PANCE Scores

5-year First Time Pass: 97%

Most Recent First Time Pass: 97%

Curriculum Structure

Didactic: 13.5 months

Clinical: 13.5 months

Rotations: 9 mandatory, 1 electives; 5 weeks each

Clinical Research Project: Required for graduation

METHODIST UNIVERSITY

Methodist University
Email: paprog@methodist.edu

5107 College Center Drive
Fayetteville, NC 28311
Phone: 910-630-7615

Mission: The mission of the Methodist University Physician Assistant Program is to establish an environment in which qualified students, recruited nationally, can develop a strong foundation in treating their patients with clinical competence, compassion and respect, while developing both personal and professional integrity.

Accreditation: Continued

Degree Offered: Master (MMS)

Start Date: August annually

Program Length: 27 months

Class Capacity: 40 students

Tuition: $82,075 (includes lab fees)

CASPA Participant: Yes

Supplemental Application: No

Admissions: Not specified

Application Deadline: January 1

GPA Requirement: None (Overall GPA of 3.0 recommended, and Prerequisite GPA 3.2 recommended)

Healthcare Experience: 500 hours required

PA Shadowing: Not required

Required Standardized Testing: GRE

Letters of Recommendation: Three required; one from a professor or advisor with the science department of your University, one from medical personnel with which you have worked in a clinical setting, and one additional letter from a professional employer or another professor, co-worker/supervisor

Seat Deposit: $1,000

Unique Program Features

PA Student Stories: You can read about current and former student stories and experiences within the program on the website.

Facilities: The program has a dedicated 8,000 square foot facility with two classrooms, nine offices, locker rooms, a kitchen, library, lounge, and clinical exam laboratory. Students also have a 7,200 square foot lecture hall and gross anatomy lab.

Inter-professional Education: At numerous times throughout didactic and clinical year students interact with Athletic Training, Health Care Administration, Kinesiology, Nursing, and Physical Therapy students.

Prerequisite Coursework

Microbiology with lab (4 credits), Anatomy and Physiology with lab (4 credits), Animal/Human Biology Courses (8 credits), General Chemistry I and II with lab (8 credits), Organic Chemistry I and II with labs (8 credits), Biochemistry (3 credits), College Algebra or higher (3 credits), Statistics (3 credits), Psychology (6 credits), Medical Terminology (1 semester). Applicants can apply with courses in progress.

UNIVERSITY OF NORTH CAROLINA

University of North Carolina
Email: paprogram@unc.edu

321 S. Columbia Street
Bondurant Hall, CB 7121
Chapel Hill, NC 27599
Phone: 919-962-8008

Mission: The mission of the University of North Carolina at Chapel Hill (UNC) Physician Assistant (PA) program is to promote high-quality, accessible, patient-centered health care for the people of North Carolina and the nation through excellence in education, scholarship, and clinical service. The UNC PA program is committed to the health care and workforce needs of North Carolinians and will use an inter-professional approach to prepare skilled and compassionate health care practitioners across the continuum of life.

Accreditation:
Provisional

Degree Offered:
Master (MHS)

Start Date:
January annually

Program Length:
24 months

Class Capacity:
20 students

Tuition:
In-state: $51,000;
Out-of-state: $95,000

CASPA Participant:
Yes

Supplemental Application: Yes

Admissions: Rolling

Application Deadline: July 1

GPA Requirement:
None (Overall GPA of 3.0 recommended, and Prerequisite GPA 3.2 recommended). Two prerequisites can be in progress but must be completed by August 31.

Healthcare Experience:
1,000 hours required

PA Shadowing: Not required

Required Standardized Testing: GRE (Scores > 150 in each section and 3.5 in writing preferred)

Letters of Recommendation:
Three required; preference is given to applicants with at least two of the three letters from experienced health care professionals who observed or supervised you in a clinical setting.

Seat Deposit: None

Prerequisite Coursework

Human Anatomy and Physiology (or Special Operations Combat Medics Course), General Biology with lab (4 credits), Microbiology (3 credits) and either General Biology II with lab or Cell Biology or Genetics or Histology or Immunology, General Chemistry with lab (4 credits) and 4 credits of General Chemistry II or Organic Chemistry or Biochemistry or Analytical Chemistry, Population Science (3 credits), Statistics or Biostatistics (3 credits). It is strongly recommended that all courses be taken in the last seven years.

No class statistics reported

PANCE Scores

5-year First Time Pass: N/A

Most Recent First Time Pass: N/A (program has not graduated first class yet)

Curriculum Structure

Didactic: 12 months

Clinical: 12 months

Rotations:
8 mandatory, 2 electives; 4-6 weeks each

Capstone Project:
Required for graduation

Unique Program Features

Non-Traditional and Veteran Focus: The program strives to provide education to non-traditional students, with attention to all veterans especially those who have served in medical military settings such as the special forces medics, for careers in medically underserved areas.

Underserved Focus: The program prepares generalist PAs to practice in rural or urban medically underserved areas through emphasis on health promotion, disease prevention, cultural competency, and primary care.

WAKE FOREST UNIVERSITY

PANCE Scores

5-year First Time Pass: 97%

Most Recent First Time Pass: 100%

Curriculum Structure

Didactic: 12 months

Clinical: 12 months

Rotations:
7 mandatory,
1 selective,
2 electives;
4 weeks each

Graduate Project:
Required for graduation

Wake Forest University
Email:
paadmit
@wakehealth.edu

Medical Center Boulevard
Winston Salem, NC 27157
Phone: 336-716-4356

Mission: We strive to produce highly capable, compassionate physician assistants who deliver patient-centered care, make significant contributions to the healthcare community, and continually advance the PA Profession. Our educators use innovative instructional methods to foster self inquiry and problem based learning, inspire an appreciation for diversity and inter-professional collaboration, and promote leadership development.

Prerequisite Coursework

Genetics (3 credits), General Chemistry or Organic Chemistry (3 credits), Biochemistry (3 credits), Anatomy and Physiology (6 credits), Microbiology with lab preferred (3 credits), Statistics (2 credits), Medical Terminology (1 course).

Accreditation: Continued

Degree Offered: Master (MMS)

Start Date: June annually

Program Length: 24 months

Class Capacity: 88 students

Tuition: $74,646

CASPA Participant: Yes

Supplemental Application: Yes

GPA Requirement: None

Healthcare Experience: 1,000 hours required

PA Shadowing: Not required

Required Standardized Testing: GRE

Letters of Recommendation: Three required; preference is given to applicants who have at least one reference from a health care professional

Seat Deposit: $750

Admissions: Rolling

Application Deadline: September 1

Unique Program Features

Inquiry-Based Learning: The curriculum is centered around inquiry-based, small-group, self-directed learning based on real patient medical problems. In inquiry-based learning (IBL), learners are progressively given more and more responsibility for their own education and become increasingly independent of the teacher for their education.

Dual Degree: The MMS-PhD is a 5- to 7-year program that combines a Master of Medical Science in Physician Assistant Studies with a PhD in Molecular Medicine and Translational Science (MMTS) and is offered in conjunction with the Wake Forest University Graduate School of Arts & Sciences. The program targets students interested in clinical research, community research, and the translation of knowledge into improved human health.

Emerging Leaders Program: The Emerging Leaders Program is a 34-month sequential degree program in which students first earn an MA in Management from the Wake Forest University School of Business (10 months) and then earn an MMS in Physician Assistant Studies within Wake Forest School of Medicine (24 months).

One Program, Two Locations: The Wake Forest PA Program is accredited for up to 64 students for the Winston-Salem campus and up to 32 students for the Boone campus.

WINGATE UNIVERSITY

Wingate University

Email: pa.wingate.edu

515 N. Main Street
PO Box 159
Wingate, NC 28170
Phone: 704-233-8993

Mission: The mission of the Wingate University Harris Department of Physician Assistant Studies is to educate physician assistant students to become competent, compassionate, and comprehensive health care providers.

Accreditation:
Continued

Degree Offered:
Master (MPAS)

Start Date:
August annually

Program Length:
27 months

Class Capacity:
50 students

Tuition: $73,000

GPA Requirement:
Prerequisite GPA 3.2

Healthcare Experience:
500 hours required

PA Shadowing: Not required

Required Standardized Testing: GRE

Letters of Recommendation: Two required; one of the letters must be from a healthcare provider (MD, DO, PA or NP)

Seat Deposit: $1,500

CASPA Participant: Yes

Supplemental Application: No

Admissions: Rolling

Application Deadline: January 15

Prerequisite Coursework

Human Anatomy and Physiology I and II with lab (8 credits), Genetics (3 credits), Microbiology with lab (4 credits), Organic Chemistry with lab (4 credits), Biochemistry (3 credits), General Psychology (3 credits), Statistics (3 credits), Medical Terminology. All science courses should be completed in 2011 or later except Organic Chemistry (no time limit). Students can apply with prerequisite courses in progress.

No class statistics reported

PANCE Scores

5-year First Time Pass: Not reported

Most Recent First Time Pass: 100%

Curriculum Structure

Didactic: 12 months

Clinical: 15 months

Rotations:
8 mandatory, 2 electives; 5 weeks each

Capstone Project:
Required for graduation

Unique Program Features

One Program, Two Locations: The Wingate Program is accredited for up to 50 students, 40 of which are placed at the Wingate campus and 10 of which are placed at the Hendersonville campus. Each campus follows the same curriculum utilizing synchronous distance learning.

NORTH DAKOTA

UNIVERSITY OF NORTH DAKOTA

University of North Dakota
Department of Physician Assistant Studies/SMHS

501 N. Columbia Road, Stop 9037
Grand Forks, ND 58202-9037
Phone: 701-777-2344
Email: und.med.paprogram
@med.und.edu

Mission: The primary mission of the University of North Dakota Physician Assistant Program is to prepare selected health care professionals to become competent physician assistants working collaboratively with physician supervision, emphasizing primary care in rural and/or underserved areas of North Dakota, the United States and the world. With this mission, the goal is to improve access to healthcare, help alleviate shortages of primary care providers and deliver comprehensive, affordable health care services to the people of rural and/or underserved populations.

Accreditation:
Continued

Degree Offered:
Master (MPAS)

Start Date:
May annually

Program Length:
24 months

Class Capacity:
35 students

Tuition:
In-state: $35,563

CASPA Participant:
Yes

Supplemental Application: Yes

Admissions: Not specified

Application Deadline:
September 1

GPA Requirement:
Overall GPA 3.0;
Prerequisite GPA 3.0

Healthcare Experience:
Track 1: Licensed/Certified Health Care Professional with minimum of 3 years experience (Registered nurse, respiratory therapist, physical therapist, radiologic technologist and paramedic). Track 2: Science-based and minimum of 500 (1000 preferred) hours of direct patient care (Certified medical assistant, certified nursing assistant, dental hygienist, emergency medical technician, and phlebotomist).

PA Shadowing: Not required

Required Standardized Testing: Not required

Letters of Recommendation: Three required; one educational, clinical, and personal letter

Seat Deposit: $200

Class of 2015
Male: not reported
Female: not reported
Minority: not reported
GPA: 3.3-3.4
Science GPA: not reported
GRE: not required
Faculty to Student Ratio: not reported
Average Healthcare Experience: not reported

PANCE Scores
5-year First Time Pass: 89%

Most Recent First Time Pass: 92%

Curriculum Structure
Students begin with 2 semesters of online basic science coursework. They then return to campus over the next year and a half for several 2-6 week sessions of didactic primary care instruction. Between didactic sessions students complete primary care clerkships and specialty clerkships. During clerkships students are responsible for additional online coursework as well.

Research Project: required for graduation

Prerequisite Coursework

Track 1: Human Anatomy (3 credits), Human Physiology (3 credits), Comprehensive Pharmacology (3 credits), Microbiology, Medical Terminology, Statistics; Track 2: Track 1 courses plus Psychology, Organic Chemistry, Biochemistry. Anatomy and Physiology should have been completed in the last 10 years and pharmacology in the last five years. All courses require a "B" or better except Organic Chemistry and Biochemistry which required a "C" or better.

Unique Program Features

Track 1 Admissions: In this track, licensed or certified healthcare providers apply as a pair with a preceptor who has agreed to precept the student on their primary care clerkships throughout the program. Preference is given to pairs that have the clinical site in rural (<25,000 population) areas and/or working with underserved populations.

Track 2 Admissions: In this track, students complete additional prerequisites and 500 hours of lower-level healthcare experience to be eligible for admissions. Students are placed by the program into their primary care clerkships and specialty clerkships. They apply as individuals.

Admissions Preference: North Dakota residents as well as residents from the surrounding states of Montana, Minnesota and South Dakota are given admissions preference, although well-qualified out of state applicants are also readily accepted.

Unique Curriculum: The didactic primary care sessions are immediately followed by a clinical practice experience, providingquick application of concepts resulting in greater development and retention of clinical competencies.

OHIO

BALDWIN WALLACE UNIVERSITY

Baldwin Wallace
University
Email:
paprogram@bw.edu

275 Eastland Road
Berea , OH 44017
Phone: 440.826.2221

Mission: Educate talented physician assistants who strive to promote the PA profession, understand the primary care workforce needs of the future, and act competently when providing excellent patient care utilizing an evidence-based and dynamic team approach.

Accreditation:
Provisional

Degree Offered:
Master (MMS)

Start Date:
May annually

Program Length:
24 months

Class Capacity:
30 students

Tuition:
$75,000 (total cost)

GPA Requirement: Overall GPA 3.0; Science GPA 3.0;

Healthcare Experience:
Preferred, not required.

PA Shadowing: Not required

Required Standardized Testing: GRE

Letters of Recommendation: Three required; one from a physician or PA, one from a college professor, and one from a manager or supervisor

Seat Deposit: $1500

CASPA Participant: Yes

Supplemental Application: Yes

Admissions: Not specified

Application Deadline:
November 1

Prerequisite Coursework

Biology I and II with lab, Anatomy and Physiology I and II with lab, Microbiology with lab, General Chemistry I and II with lab, Organic Chemistry I with lab, Introductory Psychology, English Composition, Statistics or Biostatistics, Medical Terminology. All must have been completed in the last seven years.

Unique Program Features

Admission Preferences: This program has a preference for previous graduates of Baldwin Wallace University as well as Ohio residents.

Leadership and Public Health Curriculum: Students take courses in healthcare leadership and public health and policy which are designed to give students the foundation to become effective leaders and understand how healthcare reform and public health policy impact PA practice.

Class of 2016

Male: not reported
Female: not reported
Minority: not reported
GPA: 3.64
Science GPA: not reported
GREVerbal: not reported
GRE Quantitative: not reported
GRE Writing: not reported
Faculty to Student Ratio: not reported
Average Healthcare Experience: not reported

PANCE Scores

5-year First Time Pass: 86%

Most Recent First Time Pass: 100%

Curriculum Structure

Didactic: 16 months
Clinical: 12 months
Rotations: Not specified
Master's Project: Required for graduation

Cuyahoga Community College

11000 West Pleasant Valley Road
Parma, OH 44130
Phone: 216-987-5266
Email: paprograms@tri-c.edu

Mission: To educate and prepare Physician Assistants to serve the health care needs of diverse communities.

Accreditation: Continued

Degree Offered: Certificate, Master (MSHS)

Start Date: August annually

Program Length: 28 months

Class Capacity: 30 students

Tuition:
In-state: $27,105;
Out-of-state: $51,097

GPA Requirement:
Overall GPA 3.0;
Science GPA 3.0;

Healthcare Experience: Preferred, not required.

PA Shadowing: Not required

Required Standardized Testing: None

Letters of Recommendation: Three required; one from a physician or PA

Seat Deposit: $0

CASPA Participant: Yes

Supplemental Application: Yes

Admissions: Non-rolling

Application Deadline: September 1

Unique Program Features

Veteran Preference: This program gives Veteran's preference during the admissions process.

Partnership: The partnership between Cuyahoga Community College and Cleveland State University allows students to enroll in both institutions simultaneously. Students complete the PA certificate at Cuyahoga and the Master's degree coursework simultaneously through Cleveland State.

Prerequisite Coursework

General Biology I and II, Human Anatomy and Physiology I and II, Microbiology, General Chemistry I and II with lab, Organic Chemistry or Introduction to Organic Chemistry and Biochemistry, General Psychology, Elementary Probability and Statistics, Medical Terminology. All must have been completed with a "B" or better within the last 10 years. Prerequisites can be in progress at time of application.

KETTERING COLLEGE

Kettering College

Email: pa@kc.edu

3737 Southern Boulevard
Kettering, OH 45429
Phone: 937-395-8638

Mission: Kettering College, born out of Adventist faith, offers graduate and undergraduate degrees in health science. Upholding Christ, the college educates students to make service a life calling and to view health as harmony with God in body, mind, and spirit.

Accreditation: Continued

Degree Offered: Master (MPAS)

Start Date: May annually

Program Length: 27 months

Class Capacity: 45 students

Tuition: $76,440

GPA Requirement: Prerequisite GPA 3.0

Healthcare Experience: Preferred, not required. 250 hours highly recommended.

PA Shadowing: Recommended, not required

Required Standardized Testing: None

Letters of Recommendation: Three required; no more than one letter should be from a professor; one should be from a health care professional if possible.

Seat Deposit: $500

CASPA Participant: Yes

Supplemental Application: Yes

Admissions: Not specified

Application Deadline: October 1

Class of 2015

Male: 27%
Female: 73%
Minority: not reported
GPA: 3.67
Prerequisite GPA: 3.71
GRE: not required
Faculty to Student Ratio: not reported
Average Healthcare Experience: not reported

PANCE Scores

5-year First Time Pass: 93%

Most Recent First Time Pass: 98%

Curriculum Structure

Didactic: 15 months

Clinical: 12 months

Rotations: 8 mandatory; 2 elective rotations; 4 weeks each

Capstone Project: Required for graduation

Prerequisite Coursework

Organic Chemistry I and II with lab (8 credits), Biochemistry lab preferred (4 credits), Human Anatomy and Physiology with lab (8 credits), Microbiology with lab (3-4 credits), Psychology (3 credits), Developmental or Abnormal Psychology (3 credits), Statistics (3 credits). There is a 10 year statue on all prerequisite science classes and statistics courses. Prerequisites may be in progress at the time of application but applicants must have completed 18 credits total with 12 science credits and 6 psychology or statistics credits.

Unique Program Features

Adventist Tradition: Students complete courses in spirituality in healing and healthcare as well as two semesters of clinical ethics in line with the college's founding principles.

Admissions Preference: Bonus consideration is awarded to students who have completed at least 7 credit hours at Kettering College.

Class of 2017

Male: 42%

Female: 58%

Minority: not reported

GPA: not reported

Prerequisite GPA: not reported

GRE: not reported

Faculty to Student Ratio: 8:1

Average Healthcare Experience: not reported

PANCE Scores

5-year First Time Pass: 93%

Most Recent First Time Pass: 98%

Curriculum Structure

Didactic: 15 months

Clinical: 12 months

Rotations: 8 mandatory, 1 elective; unspecified duration

LAKE ERIE COLLEGE

Lake Erie College
Email:
paeducation@lec.edu

391 W. Washington Street
Painesville, OH 44077
Phone: 855-467-8676

Mission: To recruit exemplary individuals from diverse backgrounds while creating an environment of academic excellence, leadership, and scholarly activity that produces culturally sensitive, caring Physician Assistants who practice evidence-based medicine and who are dedicated to serving the healthcare needs of the community.

Accreditation: Provisional

Degree Offered: Master (MPAS)

Start Date: May annually

Program Length: 27 months

Class Capacity: 26 students

Tuition: $72,800

CASPA Participant: Yes

Supplemental Application: No

Admissions: Rolling

Application Deadline: December 1

GPA Requirement: Overall GPA 3.2; Science GPA 3.2; Prerequisite GPA 3.0

Healthcare Experience: 250 hours required.

PA Shadowing: 50 hours required.

Required Standardized Testing: GRE

Letters of Recommendation: Three required; one from a PA, MD or DO; one from a college or university professor holding a doctorate degree; one of your choosing.

Seat Deposit: $1000

Unique Program Features

Early Clinical Exposure: Students experience early clinical experiences starting within the first several weeks of the didactic training phases. Students experience several off-site clinical experiences including: Coroner's Office, Psychiatric Clinic and Genetics Laboratory.

Integrated Educational Experience: The program provides a holistic education by utilizing faculty from other institution programs to provide course content on entrepreneurship, molecular genetics, biomedical ethics, art therapy, and counseling.

Student Biographies: Class of 2016 and 2017 student profiles are provided on the website so that applicants can get a sense of the type of student that is typically accepted.

Prerequisite Coursework

Human Anatomy and Physiology with lab (2 courses), Microbiology with lab (1 course), Genetics (1 course), General Chemistry I and II with lab (2 courses), Organic Chemistry with lab (1 course), Biology I and II with lab (2 courses), Statistics (1 course), Psychology (1 course), English (2 courses), College Algebra (1 course). All science and statistics prerequisites should have been completed in last 7 years. All courses required a "B" or higher except organic chemistry which requires a "C". Prerequisites can be in progress at time of application.

MARIETTA COLLEGE

Marietta College
Email:
paprog@marietta.edu

215 Fifth Street
Marietta, OH 45750
Phone: 740-376-4458

Mission: The mission of the Marietta College Physician Assistant Program is to help meet the need for qualified health care providers. The program accomplishes this by selecting individuals who have the academic, clinical and interpersonal aptitudes necessary for education as physician assistants.

Accreditation:
Continued

Degree Offered:
Master (MSPAS)

Start Date:
June annually

Program Length:
26 months

Class Capacity:
36 students

Tuition: $75,396

GPA Requirement:
Prerequisite GPA 3.0

Healthcare Experience:
Preferred, not required

PA Shadowing: Not required

Required Standardized Testing: GRE

Letters of Recommendation: Three required; no one specific

Seat Deposit: $500

CASPA Participant: Yes

Supplemental Application: No

Admissions: Rolling

Application Deadline:
November 1

Prerequisite Coursework

Human or Mammalian Upper Level Biology (3 credits), General Chemistry I and II with labs (4 credits), Microbiology with lab (3 credits), Human Anatomy and Physiology (6 credits), Psychology (6 credits), Statistics (3 credits). Prerequisites should be completed by fall semester prior to beginning the program, though applicants with one prerequisite in progress during spring will be considered. All courses must have been completed in the last 10 years.

Unique Program Features

Medical Mission Trips: 15 second year PA students are going to Bolivia for a medical mission trip. The students organized the trip themselves and this will be the second opportunity students have taken to visit underserved countries.

Community Service: Students routinely participate in community service opportunities including events such as 5k runs, food drives to benefit local food pantries, Relay for Life, and bone marrow drives.

Student Biographies: Class of 2016 and 2017 student profiles are provided on the website so that applicants can get a sense of the type of student that is typically accepted.

Class of 2017
Male: 22%
Female: 78%
Minority:
not reported
GPA: not reported
Prerequisite GPA:
not reported
GRE: not reported
Faculty to Student Ratio: not reported
Average Healthcare Experience:
not reported

PANCE Scores

5-year First Time Pass:
94%

Most Recent First Time Pass: 97%

Curriculum Structure
Didactic: 12 months
Clinical: 14 months
Rotations:
9 mandatory,
2 elective; 5 weeks for mandatory and 4 weeks for elective rotations
Capstone Project:
Required for graduation

No class statistics reported

PANCE Scores

5-year First Time Pass: N/A (only one year of data available)

Most Recent First Time Pass: 98%

Curriculum Structure

Didactic: 15 months

Clinical: 12 months

Rotations: 9 mandatory, 2 elective; 4 weeks each

Marietta College
Email: paprog@marietta.edu

215 Fifth Street
Marietta, OH 45750
Phone: 740-376-4458

Mission: Ohio Dominican's Physician Assistant Studies Program will educate students to become well-qualified, competent physician assistants practicing in physician supervised primary care and specialty patient focused teams. The ODU PA Program embraces a holistic approach to the pursuit of excellence in academics, research, clinical practice and community service

Unique Program Features

Admissions Preference: Preference is given to current Ohio residents, graduates of Ohio Dominican University, past or present members of the armed forces, and those with significant health care experience.

Facilities: The state-of-the-art PA program building includes cadaver labs, simulation labs, wet labs, science classrooms, collaboration rooms, and a student lounge.

Accreditation: Provisional

Degree Offered: Master (MSPAS)

Start Date: August annually

Program Length: 27 months

Class Capacity: 50 students

Tuition: $75,858

GPA Requirement: Overall GPA 3.0; Science GPA 3.0

Healthcare Experience: 250 hours.

PA Shadowing: Preferred, not required.

Required Standardized Testing: GRE

Letters of Recommendation: Two required; it is recommended at least one letter be from a clinician working in healthcare

Seat Deposit: $1500

CASPA Participant: Yes

Supplemental Application: No

Admissions: Not specified

Application Deadline: November 1

Prerequisite Coursework

Inorganic/General Chemistry with lab (4 credits), Organic Chemistry with lab (4 credits), Biochemistry (3 credits), Human Anatomy and Physiology (6 credits), Microbiology with lab (4 credits), General Biology I and II (6 credits), Intro to Psychology (3 credits), Additional Upper Level Psychology (3 credits), College Algebra or Higher Mathematics (3 credits), Statistics (3 credits), Humanities (12 credits). Courses may be in progress at time of application.

OHIO UNIVERSITY

Ohio University
Email:
painfo@ohio.edu

6805 Bobcat Way
Division of Physician Assistant Practice
Dublin, OH 43016
Phone: 614-793-3040

Class of 2017
Male: not reported
Female: not reported
Minority:
not reported
GPA: 3.45
Science GPA: 3.42
GRE Verbal:
144-166 (range)
GRE Quantitative: 144-164 (range)
GRE Writing: 3.0-5.0 (range)
Faculty to Student Ratio: not reported
Average Healthcare Experience:
not reported

PANCE Scores
5-year First Time Pass: N/A
Most Recent First Time Pass: N/A (have not graduated a class yet)

Curriculum Structure
Didactic: 15 months
Clinical: 12 months
Rotations:
9 mandatory,
1 specialty selective, 2 general selectives;
4 weeks each.
Master's Graduate Project: Required for graduation

Mission: The mission of the Ohio University Master of Physician Assistant Practice Program is to prepare students to be leaders in physician assistant practice in any clinical setting with a particular emphasis on primary care in urban and rural underserved communities in the state of Ohio and throughout Appalachia using an inter-professional team approach.

Accreditation:
Provisional

Degree Offered:
Master (MPAP)

Start Date:
May annually

Program Length:
27 months

Class Capacity:
45 students

Tuition:
$55,000 + 2,090
if non-Ohio resident

GPA Requirement:
Overall GPA 3.0;
Science GPA 3.0

Healthcare Experience:
Required, no specific number of hours

PA Shadowing: Not required

Required Standardized Testing: GRE

Letters of Recommendation: Two required; one from a physician or PA

Seat Deposit: $1000

CASPA Participant: Yes

Supplemental Application: Yes

Admissions: Non-rolling

Application Deadline:
August 1

Prerequisite Coursework

Human Anatomy and Physiology with lab (7-8 credits), Biology with lab (8 credits), Microbiology with lab (3-4 credits), General Chemistry with lab (8 credits), Organic Chemistry with lab (4 credits), Biochemistry (3 credits), Statistics (3 credits), College Algebra or higher (3 credits), General Psychology (1 course), Abnormal/Developmental/Physiological Psychology (1 course), Medical Terminology (2 credits or completion of an online module/course). Two courses can be in progress at the time of application and all science courses, statistics, and medical terminology must have been completed in the last 10 years.

Unique Program Features

Admissions Preference: The OU PA Program is actively seeking candidates who are residents of Appalachia regions of Ohio. The OU PA Program is also recruiting US Military Active Duty, National Guard, Reserve and / or Veterans. Special consideration will be given to these candidates.

Underserved Focus: In keeping with the mission of Ohio University, students enrolled in the OUPA Program will complete a portion of their clinical training in medically underserved areas of Ohio.

PANCE Scores

5-year First Time Pass: N/A

Most Recent First Time Pass: N/A (have not graduated a class yet)

Curriculum Structure

Didactic: 15 months

Clinical: 12 months

Rotations: 8 mandatory, 1 elective; range from 4-6 weeks each.

Capstone Project: Required for graduation

Unique Program Features

Facilities: State-of-the-art facilities include a student resource room and lounge, small group classrooms, mock examination rooms, and several simulation rooms. Rooms are equipped with latest technology to maximize use of devices including tablets.

UNIVERSITY OF DAYTON

University of Dayton
Email: paprogram@udayton.edu

300 College Park
Dayton, OH 45469
Phone: 937-299-2900

Mission: The PA Department's mission is to produce Physician Assistants who are committed to the service of the human person through the compassionate, ethical, and skillful provision of health care within the context of the Marianist Catholic tradition. We emphasize excellent generalist care for the whole person, particularly upholding dignity for society's most vulnerable, in a learning environment which emphasizes leadership, life-long learning, and service.

Accreditation: Provisional

Degree Offered: Master (MPAP)

Start Date: August annually

Program Length: 27 months

Class Capacity: 40 students

Tuition: $77,770

CASPA Participant: Yes

Supplemental Application: No

Admissions: Not specified

Application Deadline: December 1

GPA Requirement: Overall GPA 3.0; Science GPA 3.0; Prerequisite GPA 3.0;

Healthcare Experience: 250 hours required, 20 hours of community service required

PA Shadowing: 20 hours required

Required Standardized Testing: None

Letters of Recommendation: Three required; at least one should be from a recent college professor and one from a health care professional who has known the applicant for at least six (6) months.

Seat Deposit: $1000

Prerequisite Coursework

Human Anatomy and Physiology with lab (8 credits), Microbiology with lab (3-4 credits), Organic Chemistry with lab (8 credits), Biochemistry lab preferred (3-4 credits), General Psychology (3 credits), Second Psychology Course (3 credits), Statistics (3-4 credits), Medical Terminology (2-3 credits). A maximum of two courses can be in progress at the time of application. All science courses must have been completed in the last 10 years.

UNIVERSITY OF FINDLAY

The University
of Findlay
Email: luke@findlay.edu

Physician Assistant Program
1000 North Main Street
Findlay, OH 45840
Phone: 419-434-4529

PANCE Scores

5-year First Time Pass:
92% (only four years
of data available)

Most Recent First Time
Pass: 100%

Mission: The Physician Assistant Program at The University of Findlay is committed to providing its students with the medical knowledge necessary for them to become ethical, competent, and compassionate health care providers who deliver superior quality health care to the community in which they practice and to communities throughout the world.

Curriculum Structure

Didactic: 16 months

Clinical: 12 months

Rotations:
7 mandatory,
1 elective;
6 weeks each.

Master's Research Project: Required for graduation

Accreditation:
Continued

Degree Offered:
Master (MPA)

Start Date:
August annually

Program Length:
28 months

Class Capacity:
18 students

Tuition: $70,399

GPA Requirement:
Overall GPA 3.0;
Science GPA 3.0;
Prerequisite GPA 3.0

Healthcare Experience:
Preferred, not required.

PA Shadowing:
Preferred, not required.

Required Standardized Testing: None

Letters of Recommendation: Three
required; no one specific

Seat Deposit: $1000

Unique Program Features

Small Class Size:
The 18 student class
allows for one-on-one
mentoring of students
by faculty and fosters
a tight knit community
for academic activities,
social activities, and
community service/
engagement.

CASPA Participant: Yes

Supplemental Application: Yes

Admissions: Not specified

Application Deadline:
October 1

Prerequisite Coursework

Human Anatomy and Physiology I and II with lab, Microbiology with lab, Human Genetics (lab recommended), General Chemistry I and II with lab, Basic Organic and Biochemistry with lab or Organic Chemistry I with lab, General Physics I with lab, Medical Terminology, Statistics or higher math, General Psychology, Sociology or Cultural Anthropology. Applicants ideally should have completed prerequisites within the last 10 years.

No class statistics reported

PANCE Scores

5-year First Time Pass: 96%

Most Recent First Time Pass: 100%

Curriculum Structure

Didactic: 15 months

Clinical: 12 months

Rotations: 8 mandatory, 2 elective rotations; 4 weeks each.

Capstone Project: Required for graduation

University of Mount Union
Email: SCARPILL@ mountunion.edu

Physician Assistant Studies Program
1972 Clark Avenue
Alliance, OH 44601
Phone: 330-823-2419

Mission: The mission of the Mount Union Physician Assistant Studies Program is to educate knowledgeable, competent, and compassionate physician assistants who provide patient care with professionalism and integrity. The curriculum focuses on: the patient as an individual, the global impact of the U.S Healthcare Delivery System, the PA role on the medical team, and the importance of life-long learning for the PA.

Accreditation: Continued

Degree Offered: Master (MSPAS)

Start Date: May annually

Program Length: 27 months

Class Capacity: 40 students

Tuition: $68,600

CASPA Participant: Yes

Supplemental Application: Yes

Admissions: Not specified

Application Deadline: October 1

GPA Requirement: Overall GPA 3.0; Science GPA 3.0; Prerequisite GPA 3.0

Healthcare Experience: Preferred, not required

PA Shadowing: 40 hours required

Required Standardized Testing: GRE (>300 preferred)

Letters of Recommendation: Three required; one from a physician or PA

Seat Deposit: $500

Unique Program Features

Admissions Preference: Up to 20% of each class may consist of prior Mount Union graduates. Additionally, students who have completed certain coursework at Mount Union may be given priority admissions provided they meet GPA requirements.

Community Service: Students participate in 5K runs, Relay for Life, coat drives, holiday fundraisers, and other service-oriented activities throughout didactic and clinical year.

Graduate Testimonials: You can read about the experiences of recent graduates in the program to get a better sense of what you can expect if you enroll in the program.

Prerequisite Coursework

English Composition (3-4 credits), General Psychology (3-4 credits), General Biology I and II with labs or upper level Biology coursework (8 credits), Anatomy and Physiology I and II with labs (8 credits), Genetics (2-4 credits), Principles of Chemistry with lab (3-4 credits), Organic Chemistry I with lab (3-4 credits), Elementary Statistics or Biostatistics (3-4 credits), Microbiology with lab (4), Medical Terminology (may be completed via examination or self-directed course). All prerequisite science and math courses should be completed in the last 10 years. Two may be in progress at time of application.

UNIVERSITY OF TOLEDO

University of Toledo
Email:
physicianassistant
@utoledo.edu

3000 Arlington Avenue
MS 1027
Toledo, OH 43614
Phone: 419-383-5408

Mission: The mission of the UT Physician Assistant Program is to provide a comprehensive didactic and clinical educational programnecessary to develop highly skilled, well-educated, primary-care-oriented PAs who are capable of providing high-quality, cost-effective, patient-centered health care services ina variety of settings.

Accreditation:
Continued

Degree Offered:
Master (MSBS)

Start Date:
August annually

Program Length:
27 months

Class Capacity:
45 students

Tuition:
In-State: $43,339;
Out-of-state:
Approximately $75,000

GPA Requirement:
Overall GPA 3.0;
Prerequisite GPA 3.0

Healthcare Experience:
Preferred, not required.

PA Shadowing:
Not required

Required Standardized Testing: None

Letters of Recommendation: Two required; no one specific.

Seat Deposit: $300

No class statistics reported

PANCE Scores
5-year First Time Pass: 95%

Most Recent First Time Pass: 87%

Curriculum Structure
Didactic: 15 months
Clinical: 12 months
Rotations:
7 mandatory,
1 elective; 4 weeks each; 1 Primary Care Preceptorship of 8 weeks duration
Scholarly Project:
Required for graduation

CASPA Participant: Yes
Supplemental Application: Yes

Admissions: Non-rolling
Application Deadline:
August 1

Unique Program Features

Admissions Preference: Current Ohio residents, graduates of The University of Toledo, non-traditional, underrepresented in medicine and those who are veterans are given some degree of preference.

Academic Medical Center: The PA program is part of the larger Academic Medical Center at the University of Toledo providing students with unparalleled resources and access to experts.

Primary Care Track: After admission, students can apply to the primary care track which typically offers some funding for tuition but also requires that students participate in a primary care mentoring program, primary care student organizations, primary care elective, and annual surveys.

Prerequisite Coursework

Human Anatomy and Physiology with recommended lab (6 credits), Inorganic or General Chemistry with lab (3 credits), Organic or Biological Chemistry (3 credits), Microbiology with lab (3 credits), Psychology (6 credits), College Algebra or Statistics or any Higher Mathematics (3 credits), Medical Terminology (1 credit or by examination or self-study). All prerequisites must have been completed in the last 8 years and must have earned a "B-" or higher.

OKLAHOMA

OKLAHOMA CITY UNIVERSITY

Oklahoma City
University PA
Program

900 NE 10th St.
Oklahoma City, OK 73104
Phone: 405-208-6260
Email: not provided

Mission: To prepare physician assistants who are competent in the art and science of medicine so that they may improve lives in the communities they serve.

Accreditation: Provisional

Degree Offered: Master (MHS)

Start Date: January annually

Program Length: 28 months

Class Capacity: 36 students

Tuition: $75,000

GPA Requirement: Undergraduate or Graduate GPA 3.0

Healthcare Experience: Not required

PA Shadowing: Recommended

Required Standardized Testing: None

Letters of Recommendation: one required; no one specific

Seat Deposit: not specified

CASPA Participant: Yes

Supplemental Application: Yes

Admissions: Not specified

Application Deadline: August 1

Prerequisite Coursework

Biological Sciences (at least 5 courses totaling 15 credits), Chemistry (at least 3 courses, one of which must be biochemistry), Psychology (2 courses). All must be completed by August 15.

PANCE Scores

5-year First Time Pass: N/A

Most Recent First Time Pass: N/A (have not graduated a class yet)

Curriculum Structure

Didactic: 12 months

Clinical: 16 months

Rotations: 13 mandatory, 0 elective, 4-8 weeks each

Unique Program Features

Business Focus: The program has several courses to familiarize students with the business of medicine including Strategic Management of Healthcare Organizations, Health Care Financial Strategies and Decision Making, Health Care Marketing and Client Satisfaction, Optimizing Third Party Payment Systems, and Medical Law and Regulation.

Charitable Clinic: Each student completes a 4 week rotation in one of the charity clinics in the Oklahoma City area as part of their clinical year.

PANCE Scores

5-year First Time Pass: 98%

Most Recent First Time Pass: 100%

Curriculum Structure

Didactic: 15 months

Clinical: 15 months

Rotations: 9 mandatory, 2 elective, 1 preceptorship, 2-8 weeks each

Capstone Project: required for graduation

Prerequisite Coursework

English Composition I and II (6 credits), College Algebra (3 credits), Psychology (6 credits), Chemistry (12 credits, at least 3 of which must be Organic Chemistry or Biochemistry), Microbiology with lab (4 credits), Upper Division Science (6 credits), Human Anatomy with lab (4 credits), Human Physiology with lab (4 credits). Anatomy, Physiology, and Upper Division Sciences must be completed within the last 7 years.

UNIVERSITY OF OKLAHOMA, TULSA

OUHSC Office of Admissions and Records
Email: outulsapa@ouhsc.edu

Basic Sciences Education Building
Room 200
Oklahoma City, OK 73126
Phone: 918-660-3842

Mission: The mission of the Physician Assistant Program at the University of Oklahoma, Tulsa School of Community Medicine, is to train physician assistants to provide quality health care to the citizens of Oklahoma with an emphasis on serving both rural and urban underserved populations.

Accreditation: Continuing

Degree Offered: Master (MHS)

Start Date: June annually

Program Length: 30 months

Class Capacity: 24 students

Tuition: In-state: $28,775; Out-of-state: $65,895

GPA Requirement: Overall GPA 2.75; Science GPA 2.75

Healthcare Experience: Preferred, not required

PA Shadowing: Not required

Required Standardized Testing: GRE

Letters of Recommendation: Three required; no one specific

Seat Deposit: $150

CASPA Participant: Yes

Supplemental Application: Yes

Admissions: Non-rolling

Application Deadline: October 1

Unique Program Features

Summer Institute: This week-long event is the hallmark of the OU Tulsa School of Community Medicine's innovative education program. The immersive experience engages participants in a curriculum of reflective, experiential service learning. Participants serve in an interdisciplinary group of both students and faculty representing colleges from across the Tulsa campus. Participants interact with community members including patients, healthcare providers and community agencies to gain an understanding of the intricacies of the healthcare community within the Tulsa area. As part of the Summer Institute, participants also experience a poverty simulation designed to create an understanding of the challenges facing many members of our community.

PA Longitudinal Clinic: This is a student experience that allows students to manage their own panel of patients, twice per month, providing a continuous care environment for chronic disease management.

UNIVERSITY OF OKLAHOMA, OKLAHOMA CITY

University of Oklahoma, Oklahoma City
Email: infookc-pa@ouhsc.edu

900 NE 10th Street
Suite 2600
Oklahoma City, OK 73104
Phone: 405-271-2058

Mission: Our mission is to attract the best talent in the region from diverse backgrounds and equip them with the capability to provide excellent patient care to the varied populations in Oklahoma and the region.

Accreditation:
Probation

Degree Offered:
Master (MHS)

Start Date:
June annually

Program Length:
30 months

Class Capacity:
50 students

Tuition:
In-state: $28,775;
Out-of-state: $65,895

GPA Requirement:
Overall GPA 2.75

Healthcare Experience:
Preferred, not required

PA Shadowing: Not required

Required Standardized Testing: GRE

Letters of Recommendation: Three required; no one specific

Seat Deposit: $150

CASPA Participant: Yes

Supplemental Application: Yes

Admissions: Non-rolling

Application Deadline:
October 1

Prerequisite Coursework

College Algebra or higher, Introduction of Psychology, Psychology elective, General Chemistry I, General Chemistry II, Physics, Human Anatomy, Human Physiology, Microbiology, Pathogenic Microbiology or Immunology or Virology or Genetics.

Unique Program Features

Rotations: All rotations are completed in Oklahoma with the exception of the elective preceptorship, limiting the required travel for students.

Volunteerism: The student society is active in volunteerism. Recently several students volunteered at the Oklahoma City Memorial Marathon, as an example.

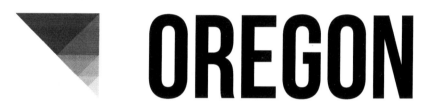

OREGON

OREGON HEALTH & SCIENCE UNIVERSITY

Oregon Health &
Science University
Email:
paprgm@ohsu.edu

2730 SW Moody Avenue
CL5PA
Portland, OR 97201
Phone: 503-494-3633

Mission: Prepare physician assistants for the practice of medicine and the delivery of primary care services to diverse populations, including the medically underserved, contribute to meeting the health workforce needs of Oregon, provide a model of excellence in physician assistant education and, promote the physician assistant profession in the state.

Accreditation:
Continuing

Degree Offered:
Master (MPAS)

Start Date:
June annually

Program Length:
26 months

Class Capacity:
42 students

Tuition: $79,947

GPA Requirement:
Overall GPA: 2.8;
Science GPA: 2.8

Healthcare Experience:
2,000 hours required

PA Shadowing: Not required

Required Standardized Testing: GRE

Letters of Recommendation: Three required; no one specific

Seat Deposit: $700

CASPA Participant: Yes

Supplemental Application: No

Admissions: Rolling

Application Deadline:
September 1

Class of 2018
Male: 27%
Female: 73%
Minority:
Not reported
GPA: 3.48
Science GPA:
not reported
GRE: not reported
Faculty to Student Ratio: not reported
Average Healthcare Experience:
not reported

PANCE Scores

5-year First Time Pass:
98%

Most Recent First Time Pass: 100%

Curriculum Structure

Didactic: 12 months

Clinical: 14 months

Rotations: 7 mandatory, 3 elective, 5 weeks each

Prerequisite Coursework

Human Anatomy and Physiology with labs (2 semesters), Microbiology with lab (3 credits), Biology (3 credits), Chemistry (8 credits), General or Developmental Psychology (3 credits), Biostatistics or Statistics (3 credits). Overall, students must have completed 30 credit hours of Biology, Chemistry and Physics and also must have completed Anatomy and Physiology within 7 years of program matriculation.

Unique Program Features

Admissions Preference: The program gives preference to residents of Oregon, Veterans, non-resident applications with Oregon Heritage, and resident and non-resident applications with superior achievements or interest/experience in rural health, underserved populations and/or primary care.

Community Outreach Project: Each student designs, implements, and evaluates a community outreach project during their clinical year on a topic of their choosing to a community group.

Rural Track: Students interested in practicing rural medicine can join the rural track and will be assigned a rotation at one of OHSU's campuses for rural health, complete a rural community based project, complete a community outreach project for the rural community, and also attend special lectures with a rural medicine focus during callback days.

Class of 2017

Male: 28%

Female: 72%

Minority: Not reported

GPA: not reported

Science GPA: 3.59

GRE: not required

Faculty to Student Ratio: not reported

Average Healthcare Experience: 3,800 hours

PANCE Scores

5-year First Time Pass: 94%

Most Recent First Time Pass: 100%

Curriculum Structure

Didactic: 13 months

Clinical: 15 months

Rotations: 7 mandatory, 2 elective, 6 weeks each

Graduate Project: required for graduation

PACIFIC UNIVERSITY

Pacific University
Email:
gradadmissions
@pacificu.edu

190 SE 8th Avenue
Suite 181
Hillsboro, OR 97123
Phone: Not provided

Mission: The School of Physician Assistant Studies prepares and mentors students within an innovative curriculum to provide quality care for a diverse global community focusing on primary care for underserved and rural populations.

Accreditation: Continuing

Degree Offered: Master (MSPAS)

Start Date: May annually

Program Length: 27 months

Class Capacity: 50 students

Tuition: $84,495

GPA Requirement:
Overall GPA: 2.75;
Science GPA: 2.75;
Prerequisite GPA 2.75

Healthcare Experience: 1,000 hours required

PA Shadowing: Not required

Required Standardized Testing: None

Letters of Recommendation: Two required; no one specific

Seat Deposit: $1,000

CASPA Participant: Yes

Supplemental Application: Yes

Admissions: Rolling

Application Deadline: September 1

Unique Program Features

Curriculum Design: The curriculum uses system-based modules. In the morning students attend traditional lectures, while in the afternoon they focus on case-based small group learning.

Unique Tracks: The program offers several different tracks depending on applicant interest include a rural healthcare track, interprofessional track, and global medicine track.

Outreach Initiatives: The program has both a Hawaii and Veterans Outreach initiative aimed to garner more student interest from these groups and giving some admissions preference to students in either category.

Prerequisite Coursework

Human Anatomy and Physiology I and II with lab, Microbiology or Bacteriology, General Chemistry I and II with labs, Organic Chemistry or Biochemistry, Statistics (3 credits), Psychology or Sociology (3 credits). All courses must be completed by December 31 of the application year.

PENNSYLVANIA

ARCADIA UNIVERSITY (2 CAMPUSES)

Arcadia University
450 S. Easton Road
Glenside, PA 19038
Phone:215-572-2888
Email: admiss
@arcadia.edu

Arcadia University
111 Continental Drive
Suite 201
Newark, DE 19713
Phone: 302-356-9440
Email:admiss@arcadia.edu

Mission: Arcadia University Physician Assistant Program is dedicated to training highly competent, globally aware physician assistants who are prepared to be life-long learners. The Program is committed to fostering excellence in patient care and promoting professionalism, leadership, cultural competency, scholarship, and service.

Accreditation:
Continuing

Degree Offered:
Master (MMS)

Start Date:
May annually

Program Length:
24 months

Class Capacity:
50 students

Tuition: $80,400

GPA Requirement:
Overall GPA 3.0;
Science GPA 3.0

Healthcare Experience:
200 hours required

PA Shadowing: Not required

Required Standardized Testing: GRE or MCAT

Letters of Recommendation: Three required; not from anyone specific

Seat Deposit: $500

CASPA Participant: Yes

Supplemental Application: No

Admissions: Rolling

Application Deadline:
December 1

Prerequisite Coursework

Biological Sciences (5 courses, to include Anatomy, Physiology, and Microbiology; Biochemistry is recommended), Chemistry (3 courses, to include at least one semester of Organic Chemistry), Psychology (1 semester), Statistics (1 semester)

Class of 2016
GPA: 3.71
Science GPA: 3.67
GRE: 310 combined verbal and quantitative, 4.12 analytical

PANCE Scores

5-year First Time Pass: 100%

Most Recent First Time Pass: 100%

Curriculum Structure

Didactic: 12 months

Clinical: 12 months

Rotations:
7 mandatory (ranging from 4-8 weeks), 3 electives (4 weeks each)

Capstone Project:
Not required

Unique Program Features

Dual Degree: Option to get a dual MPH or Masters in Health education.

Pre-PA Track: 4+2 track available for incoming undergraduates.

Rotations: International rotations available.

Community Service: One-week medical mission trips in Panama and Nicaragua are offered to students.

PANCE Scores

5-year First Time Pass: 95%

Most Recent First Time Pass: 100%

Curriculum Structure

Didactic: 12 months

Clinical: 12 months

Rotations: 7 mandatory, 2 elective

Capstone Project: Not required

Unique Program Features

None reported

Prerequisite Coursework

General Biology I and II with lab (2 semesters), General (Inorganic) Chemistry I and II with lab (2 semesters), Anatomy with lab (1 semester), Physiology (1 semester), Microbiology (1 semester), General Psychology (1 semester), English (1 semester), Medical Terminology (1 semester) All prerequisites must be completed with a "B" or better. All courses must be completed by June 1st prior to the August matriculation.

CHATHAM UNIVERSITY

Chatham University

Email: GradAdmissions@ Chatham.edu

MPAS Program, Office of Graduate Admissions, Berry Hall Woodland Road Pittsburgh, PA 15232 Phone:412-365-2988

Mission: To strive for excellence in physician assistant education whose graduates are known as outstanding clinicians in the community and leaders in the profession trained by faculty who are recognized for developing and researching innovative curricular methods. The Chatham University MPAS Program is dedicated to producing knowledgeable, compassionate, ethical, and clinically skillful graduates that are ready to provide health care services to all persons without exclusion and who are willing to become the future leaders and educators of the profession.

Accreditation: Continuing

Degree Offered: Master (MPAS)Start Date: August annually

Program Length: 24 months

Class Capacity: 80 students

Tuition: $102,686

CASPA Participant: Yes

Supplemental Application: No

Admissions: Not reported

Application Deadline: October 1

GPA Requirement: Overall GPA 3.25; Science GPA 3.25

Healthcare Experience: Not required

PA Shadowing: Required (8 hours)

Required Standardized Testing: GRE

Letters of Recommendation: Three required; One academic letter, one from a volunteer or work supervisor, and one letter at the applicant's discretion

Seat Deposit: $600

DESALES UNIVERSITY

Desales University

Email:
mspas@desales.edu

Physician Assistant Program
2755 Station Avenue
Center Valley, PA 18034
Phone: 610 282-1415

Class Statistics
Faculty to Student
Ratio: 1:12

PANCE Scores
5-year First Time Pass:
100%

Most Recent First Time
Pass: 100%

Curriculum Structure
Didactic: 12 months
Clinical: 12 months
Rotations:
8 mandatory,
1 elective
Capstone Project:
Not required

Mission: The mission of the Physician Assistant program is consistent with the enduring Christian Humanistic traditions of DeSales University and seeks to graduate physician assistants who dedicate themselves to the patient as an individual. Physician assistant graduates will further the vision of Christian Humanism and Salesian tradition by: focusing on preventative health care and wellness; promoting competent and capable health care to patients of diverse populations in a variety of settings; emphasizing the patient holistically, i.e., considering the context of family, local community, and society in general; promoting life-long learning; supporting cultural diversity; and incorporating ethical principles into a patient-focused practice.

Accreditation:
Continuing
Degree Offered:
Master (MSPAS)
Start Date:
August annually
Program Length:
24 months
Class Capacity:
80 students
Tuition: $73,950

CASPA Participant:
Yes

Supplemental Application: No

Admissions: Rolling

Application Deadline: December 1

GPA Requirement: Overall GPA 3.0; Science GPA 3.0

Healthcare Experience:500 hours required

PA Shadowing: Recommended

Community Service:
Preference is given to individuals with at least 100 hours of community service or volunteer work.

Required Standardized Testing: None

Letters of Recommendation: Three required; not from anyone specific

Seat Deposit: $500

Prerequisite Coursework

Human Anatomy & Physiology I and II , English Composition I and II , General Biology, Inorganic Chemistry, Microbiology, Organic Chemistry, Psychology, Statistics

Anatomy and Physiology as well as Microbiology must have been taken within five years of applying to the program; exceptions may be considered for applicants who have been active in the medical field since taking the course.

Unique Program Features

Pre-PA Track: 3+2 option for undergraduates (Medical Studies major).

Curriculum: Participation in the Free Clinic is part of the curriculum for all students. The clinic is open two evenings per week and provides completely free primary and acute care, laboratory services and medications to the men seeking shelter or enrolled in a recovery program at the Allentown Rescue Mission.

Facilities: The Gambet center is a new 77,000 sq. ft., $27 million facility that includes state-of-the-science simulation laboratories to replicate clinical scenarios specific to adult, pediatric and birthing care for undergraduate and graduate health care degree programs. Desales also has simulation training labs.

Rotations: Students have the opportunity to complete their elective rotation abroad in Manchay, Peru.

DREXEL UNIVERSITY

No class statistics reported

PANCE Scores

5-year First Time Pass: 97%

Most Recent First Time Pass: 97%

Curriculum Structure

Didactic: 12 months

Clinical: 15 months

Rotations: 8 mandatory (six are 5 weeks long and two primary care rotations are 10 weeks long)

Graduate Project: Required for graduation

Unique Program Features

Academics: Part-time option available to be completed in 3 years. The didactic year is split into 2 years and the clinical year is completed the same as the full-time program in year 3.

Drexel University
Email:
paadmissions
@drexel.edu

3 Parkway
1601 Cherry Street, 6th Floor, MS#6504
Philadelphia, PA 19102
Phone:267-359-5758

Mission: Educate primary care physician assistants, improve health care delivery in rural and urban medically underserved areas, and promote the physician assistant profession.

Accreditation: Continuing

Degree Offered: Master (MHS)

Start Date: September annually

Program Length: 27 months

Class Capacity: 75 students

Tuition: $81,666

CASPA Participant: Yes

Supplemental Application: No

Admissions: Rolling

Application Deadline: October 1

GPA Requirement: Overall GPA 3.0; Science GPA 3.0

Healthcare Experience: 500 hours required

PA Shadowing: Recommended

Community Service: Preference is given to individuals with at least 100 hours of community service or volunteer work.

Required Standardized Testing: None

Letters of Recommendation: Three required; not from anyone specific

Seat Deposit: $500

Prerequisite Coursework

Human Anatomy & Physiology with lab (2 semesters), General Biology with lab (2 semesters), General Chemistry with lab (1 semester), Microbiology (1 semester), Psychology (1 semester), Genetics (1 semester), Medical Terminology (1 semester). All prerequisites must be completed with a grade of "B-" or better. It is encouraged that all prerequisite courses are completed before applying.

DUQUESNE UNIVERSITY

Duquesne University
Email:
admissions@duq.edu

600 Forbes Avenue
Pittsburgh, PA 15282
Phone: 412-396-5914

Mission: The mission of the Duquesne University Physician Assistant Studies Program is four-fold: to prepare trainees with the necessary knowledge and skills to reliably perform the role of a physician assistant; to promote a lifelong responsibility for ongoing learning and active participation in a changing health care environment; to instill a professional identity in each student based on the education for the mind, heart and spirit that is achieved at Duquesne; to prepare graduates to provide quality primary health care among rural, urban and minority populations.

Accreditation:
Continuing

Degree Offered:
Master (MPAS)

Start Date:
May annually

Program Length:
27 months

Class Capacity:
40 students

Tuition:
$222,678 (entire undergraduate and masters program)

CASPA Participant: No

Supplemental Application: No

Admissions: Rolling; option for early action

Application Deadline:
December 1

GPA Requirement:
3.0 overall high school GPA

Healthcare Experience:
Not required

PA Shadowing:
Recommended in order to gain an understanding of the PA profession, but no specific number of hours required

Required Standardized Testing: SAT or ACT; a composite math and verbal SAT score of at least 1,100 or a composite ACT score of at least 24

Letters of Recommendation: One required (from an academic source such as a teacher or counselor)

Seat Deposit: $500

No class statistics reported

PANCE Scores
5-year First Time Pass: 92%

Most Recent First Time Pass: 96%

Curriculum Structure

Didactic: 14 months (following three years of undergraduate core science coursework)

Clinical: 12 months

Rotations:
7 mandatory,
1 elective
(all 6 weeks long)

Evidence Based Medicine Master's Project: Required for graduation

Unique Program Features

Program: First five-year, entry-level Master's degree program in the nation. "Entry level" students come into Duquesne University as freshmen, complete the five year curriculum, and earn both a Bachelor of Science in Health Sciences degree and a Master of Physician Assistant Studies degree.

Prerequisite Coursework

Since students apply in high school, the only prerequisites for applying are advanced science and math coursework (minimum of 7 units), demonstration of leadership skills, involvement in extracurricular activities, and demonstration of knowledge of the PA profession.

PANCE Scores

5-year First Time Pass: 91%

Most Recent First Time Pass: 95%

Curriculum Structure

Didactic: 4 years (combined undergraduate and PA didactic)

Clinical: 12 months

Rotations: 6 mandatory, 2 elective (all 6 weeks long)

Capstone Project: Research proposal required for graduation

Unique Program Features

Program: This program is primarily a 5-year program starting at the undergraduate level. They currently don't have any seats available for post-baccalaureate applicants.

GANNON UNIVERSITY

Gannon University
Email: schlick001@gannon.edu

109 University Square
Erie, PA 16541
Phone: 800-426-6668

Mission: The Gannon University Physician Assistant Program strives to provide a stimulating learning environment, highly qualified and motivated faculty, as well as modern facilities that offer Physician Assistant students the opportunity to become well-prepared primary care providers who are leaders in their field and community.

Accreditation: Continuing

Degree Offered: Masters (MPAS)

Start Date: August annually

Program Length: 44 months

Class Capacity: 58 students

Tuition: $180,365 (5-year program)

GPA Requirement: Overall GPA 3.2

Healthcare Experience: 30 hours required

PA Shadowing: Not required

Required Standardized Testing: SAT score of 1050 or ACT score of 23

Letters of Recommendation: Three required; One from a counselor

Seat Deposit: $300

CASPA Participant: No

Supplemental Application: No

Admissions: Not reported, but very competitive so early application is advised

Application Deadline: November 1 (senior year of high school)

Prerequisite Coursework

Completion of 16 academic units at the high school level, four of which must be English; four in social sciences, at least two units of math, including algebra, both with Bs or higher. Two to four units of science including biology and chemistry with labs and grades of Bs or higher.

KING'S COLLEGE

King's College

Email:
PAadmissions@kings.edu

133 North River Street
Wilkes-Barre, PA 18612
Phone: 570-208-5853

Mission: The mission of the King's College Department of Physician Assistant Studies is to provide students with a primary care-based foundation of knowledge, technical skills, critical thinking, and moral values to become competent and cost-effective healthcare providers.

Accreditation:
Continuing

Degree Offered:
Master of Science in
PA Studies

Start Date:
August annually

Program Length:
24 months

Class Capacity:
67 students

Tuition:
$78,900; $176,820
for the 5-year
combined program

GPA Requirement:
Overall GPA 3.2;
Science GPA 3.2

Healthcare Experience:
500 hours required

PA Shadowing: Required
(no specific number of hours);
counted towards healthcare
experience

**Required Standardized
Testing:** None

**Letters of
Recommendation:** Two
required; not from anyone
specific

Seat Deposit: $750

CASPA Participant: Yes

**Supplemental
Application:** No

Admissions: Rolling

Application Deadline:
October 1

Class of 2014
GPA: 3.67
Science GPA: 3.61

PANCE Scores
5-year First Time Pass:
94%

Most Recent First Time
Pass: 98%

**Curriculum
Structure**
Didactic:
10.5 months

Clinical: 13.5 months

Rotations:
8 mandatory,
1 elective
(all 6 weeks long)

Capstone Project:
Required for
graduation

**Unique Program
Features**

Pre-PA Track: Offer a
combined 5-year BS/MS
program.

Facilities: New state
of the art multimedia
facilities with new
cadaver lab.

Prerequisite Coursework

Anatomy and Physiology I and II (2 semesters), General Biology (2 semesters), Chemistry (2 semesters), Microbiology (1 semester). Prerequisite courses should be completed preferably with labs. Prerequisites cannot be taken online. Candidates cannot have any outstanding courses in the summer prior to the start of the program in August.

Class of 2014

Male: 28%
Female: 72%
Minority: Not reported
GPA: 3.55
Science GPA: 3.43
GRE: Verbal 153, Quantitative 154, Writing 4.1
Faculty to Student Ratio: Not reported
Average Healthcare Experience: Not reported

PANCE Scores

5-year First Time Pass: 96%

Most Recent First Time Pass: 96%

Curriculum Structure

Didactic: 12 months
Clinical: 12 months
Rotations: 3 blocks of clerkships; rotations are typically 6 weeks long and are concentrated in the areas of behavioral and mental health, pediatrics, obstetrics, gynecology, emergency medicine, general internal medicine, and general surgery. There is an 18-week primary care preceptorship.
Capstone Project: Not required

LOCK HAVEN UNIVERSITY

Lock Haven University Physician Assistant Program

401 N. Fairview Street
Lock Haven, PA 17745
Phone: 570-484-2929
Email: paportal@lhup.edu

Mission: The mission of the program is to educate highly-skilled Physician Assistants who: are capable of providing quality health care; have expertise in the health care needs of the medically underserved; are prepared to critically evaluate, and become leaders in bringing about improvement in the medical and social systems that affect the health of underserved populations; will seek and retain employment as primary care Physician Assistants in medically underserved areas of the Commonwealth of Pennsylvania.

Accreditation: Continuing
Degree Offered: Master (MHS)
Start Date: May annually
Program Length: 24 months
Class Capacity: 72 students
Tuition: $53,736 (in-state); $76,874 (out-of-state)

GPA Requirement: Overall GPA 3.0; Science GPA 3.0; Prerequisite GPA 3.0
Healthcare Experience: Preferred/Recommended
PA Shadowing: Not required
Required Standardized Testing: GRE
Letters of Recommendation: Three required; not from anyone specific
Seat Deposit: $500

CASPA Participant: Yes
Supplemental Application: No

Admissions: Not reported
Application Deadline: October 1

Prerequisite Coursework

General Chemistry I and II (2 semesters), Biology or Zoology (2 semesters), Human Anatomy and Physiology (2 semesters), Microbiology (1 semester), Human Genetics (1 semester), Statistics (1 semester) All prerequisite courses must be completed with a grade "B" or better.

Unique Program Features

Multiple Campuses: The Lock Haven program has expanded and now offers PA education at its Clearfield, Coudersport, and Harrisburg campuses.

Pre-PA Track: Option for 3+2 combined BS/MHS program for incoming undergraduates.

Scholarship: Some scholarships are available through numerous benefactors of the Lock Haven University Physician Assistant Program.

MARYWOOD UNIVERSITY

Marywood University
Email:
paprogram@marywood.edu

2300 Adams Avenue
Scranton, PA 18509
Phone: 570-348-6298

Mission: The Physician Assistant (PA) Program at Marywood University is committed to providing students with an exceptional education in a supportive and nurturing environment. This professional education includes the knowledge necessary to diagnose, treat, educate and empower patients in a variety of settings across the lifespan. We acknowledge that every patient is more than just their physical body, therefore our program is dedicated to teaching our students the appreciation of the patients' spirit as well as caring for their body. There is an emphasis on the importance of sharing knowledge with future PA students while providing leadership within the community while promoting the PA profession. Every student will develop as both a professional and as a leader throughout their educational career within this program. Marywood University's PA Program has an awareness of the need for quality healthcare, both regionally and globally, as each student is prepared to deal with the changing health care environment.

No class statistics reported

PANCE Scores
5-year First Time Pass: 88%

Most Recent First Time Pass: 88%

Curriculum Structure
- **Didactic:** 12 months
- **Clinical:** 15 months
- **Rotations:** 7 mandatory, 1 elective (ranging from 6-12 weeks)
- **Capstone Project:** Not required

Accreditation: Continuing

Degree Offered: Master of PA Studies

Start Date: May annually

Program Length: 27 months

Class Capacity: 45 students

Tuition: $57,275

GPA Requirement: Overall GPA 3.0; Science GPA 3.0

Healthcare Experience: 500 hours

PA Shadowing: Recommended

Required Standardized Testing: GRE

Letters of Recommendation: Three required; not from anyone specific

Seat Deposit: $500

CASPA Participant: Yes
Supplemental Application: No

Admissions: Not reported

Application Deadline: November 1

Prerequisite Coursework

General Chemistry with lab (2 semesters), Organic Chemistry with lab (2 semesters), General Biology with lab (2 semesters), Microbiology with lab (1 semester), Anatomy and Physiology with lab (2 semesters), Medical Terminology (1 course)

Unique Program Features

Pre-PA Track: Students in the pre-professional phase are required to maintain an overall GPA of 3.00, as well as a 3.00 average in all prerequisite science courses and/or labs to be considered for admission to the professional phase. Students who have successfully met all required liberal arts core requirements and science prerequisites may apply for admission to the professional program, following their second year as Pre-PA.

Clinical Tracks: Unique to Marywood's PA Program, students may choose to focus their studies and clinical experience by applying for acceptance to one the following Clinical Tracks during the clinical phase of the program: Emergency Medicine, Orthopedics/Sports Medicine, Pediatrics, Hospitalist, General Surgery.

Facilities: Newly renovated Physical Assessment Lab that includes 22 exam tables and 5 private exam rooms for practical education and individual testing of history taking and physical examination techniques. In addition, there are X-ray view boxes, operating room scrub sinks and a variety of teaching models.

MERCYHURST UNIVERSITY

Mercyhurst University
Email:
srogers@mercyhurst.edu

501 East 38th Street
Erie, PA 16546
Phone: 814-824-2598

Mission: The mission of the Department of Physician Assistant Studies (DPAS) is to prepare students with the highest quality academic and clinical training. The program will prepare physician assistants to be leaders in the profession, proficient in meeting the challenges of healthcare, while providing compassionate, quality care to the diverse communities in which they serve. The department's mission, vision and core goals were developed to align with the university's mission, vision and core values. Emphasis has been placed on the Mercy tradition and healthcare core values to stay true to the basic principles set forth by our founders.

Accreditation: Continuing

Degree Offered: Master (MSPAS)

Start Date: June annually

Program Length: 24 months

Class Capacity: 25 students

Tuition: $74,981

GPA Requirement: Overall GPA 3.2; Prerequisite GPA 3.2

Healthcare Experience: 200 hours required

PA Shadowing: Not required

Required Standardized Testing: GRE

Letters of Recommendation: Three required; not from anyone specific

Seat Deposit: $600

CASPA Participant: Yes

Supplemental Application: Yes

Admissions: Not reported

Application Deadline: December 1

Prerequisite Coursework

Biology with lab (2 semesters), Chemistry with lab (General and Organic, 3 semesters), Biochemistry with lab (1 semester), Anatomy with lab (1 semester), Physiology with lab (1 semester), Microbiology with lab (1 semester), Genetics (1 semester), Statistics (1 semester), Psychology (1 semester), Nutrition (1 semester), Medical Terminology (1 course)

MISERICORDIA UNIVERSITY

Misericordia University
Email: paadmissions @misericordia.edu

301 Lake Street
Dallas, PA 18612
Phone: 570-674-6716

No class statistics provided

PANCE Scores
No scores available yet

Curriculum Structure

Didactic: 12 months

Clinical: 12 months

Rotations:
8 mandatory,
1 elective,
5 weeks each

Thesis Project:
required for graduation

Mission: The mission of the Misericordia University Physician Assistant program is to provide opportunities for exceptional students to acquire the highest quality cognitive education and training experience in an atmosphere of academic excellence. Graduates will achieve their maximum potential as able, caring, compassionate, competent, idealistic professionals. The program's educational environment will promote an ethos of service, responsibility, morals and ethics, a quest for excellence, and an avid desire for self-directed lifelong learning in a spiritually enriched environment, while preparing students to apply evidence-based knowledge. Program graduates will exhibit honesty, communication skills, talents, dedication, self-discipline, initiative, resourcefulness, and judgment as collaborating clinical practitioners. Graduates will be dedicated to their patients and communities, showing respect for the dignity, worth, and rights of others, while serving with integrity, accountability, and trust as leaders in an evolving profession, and as advocates and innovators dedicated to augmenting, complementing, and advancing the quality, accessibility, and transformation of the healthcare system.

Unique Program Features

Community Service: The program's students are very active and complete several projects each year.

Facilities: The program offers both an anatomy lab and simulation lab to students.

Accreditation:
Provisional

Degree Offered:
Master (MSPAS)

Start Date:
August annually

Program Length:
24 months

Class Capacity:
20 students

Tuition: $83,011

GPA Requirement:
GPAOverall GPA 3.0;
Science GPA 3.0;
Prerequisite GPA 3.0

Healthcare Experience:
200 hours required

PA Shadowing: Not required

Required Standardized Testing: GRE

Letters of Recommendation: Three required; not from anyone specific

Seat Deposit: $750

Prerequisite Coursework

Biology with lab (8 credits), General and Organic Chemistry with labs (12 credits), Biochemistry with lab (4 credits), Anatomy with lab (4 credits), Physiology with lab (4 credits), Microbiology with lab (4 credits), Genetics (3 credits), Statistics (3 credits), Psychology (3 credits), Nutrition (3 credits), Medical Terminology (1 credits). Physiology and Microbiology must be completed within 5 years of matriculation.

CASPA Participant: Yes

Supplemental Application: No

Admissions: Rolling

Application Deadline: December 1

Class of 2017

Male: 63%

Female: 37%

Minority: 47%

GPA: 3.63

Science GPA: 3.69

GRE: Total – 313;
Verbal – 158;
Quantitative – 155;
Writing – 4.2

Faculty to Student Ratio: Not reported

Average Healthcare Experience:
6,522 hours

PANCE Scores

No scores available yet

Curriculum Structure

Didactic: 12 months

Clinical: 12 months

Rotations:
8 mandatory,
1 elective (all 5 weeks)

Capstone Project:
Not required

PENN STATE UNIVERSITY

Penn State College of Medicine
Email: psupaprogram @hmc.psu.edu

Physician Assistant Program, Mail Code H152
500 University Drive
Hershey, PA 17033
Phone: 717-531-0003 (ext. 285595)

Mission: The Physician Assistant (PA) Program's mission is to prepare graduates to be academically, clinically, professionally, and culturally competent in the delivery of health care services, to develop critical thinking and application skills, and to provide compassionate and comprehensive care to the patients that they will serve. Our graduates will improve the health of their patients and the populations that they serve in an efficient and cost-conscious manner.

Accreditation:
Provisional

Degree Offered:
Master (MPAS)

Start Date:
May annually

Program Length:
24 months

Class Capacity:
30 students

Tuition: $73,504

GPA Requirement: Overall GPA 3.0; Science GPA 3.0;

Healthcare Experience:
500 hours required

PA Shadowing:
Not required

Required Standardized Testing: GRE or MCAT

Letters of Recommendation: Three required; not from anyone specific

Seat Deposit: $500

CASPA Participant: Yes

Supplemental Application: Yes (no fee)

Admissions: Not reported

Application Deadline:
January 15

Unique Program Features

Facilities: Students in the Penn State PA program have full use of the 10,000 square foot simulation center and clinical skills laboratories. Additionally, the program will have a clinical anatomy with full cadaver dissection as part of pre-clinical training.

Team-Based Learning: The program offers this unique style where students work as teams to solve clinical problems and learn didactic information.

Prerequisite Coursework

General Biology (1 semester), Anatomy and Physiology (2 semesters), Microbiology (1 semester), General or Principles of Chemistry (1 semester), Biochemistry or Organic Chemistry (1 semester), General Psychology (1 semester), Statistics or Biostatistics (1 semester), English Composition (2 semesters)

PENNSYLVANIA COLLEGE OF TECHNOLOGY

Pennsylvania College of Technology

Physician Assistant Program
Dif 123, One College Avenue
Williamsport, PA 17701
Phone: 570-327-4779

Mission: The School of Health Sciences at Pennsylvania College of Technology is committed to preparing professional and competent practitioners. Our programs are structured to support and develop essential qualities of caring, accountability, a credible work ethic, critical thinking, information literacy, and effective interpersonal skills to address social demands. Graduates will be prepared to enter the health professions workforce and be eligible for licensure, certification, and advanced education.

Accreditation: Continuing

Degree Offered: BS in Physician Assistant

Start Date: August annually

Program Length: 24 months

Class Capacity: 30 students

Tuition: $15,810 per semester (in-state); $22,470 per semester (out-of-state)

GPA Requirement: Overall GPA 3.0; Science GPA 3.0; Prerequisite GPA 3.0

Healthcare Experience: 300 hours required

PA Shadowing: Required (16 hours)

Required Standardized Testing: None

Letters of Recommendation: No

Seat Deposit: None

CASPA Participant: No

Supplemental Application: No

Admissions: Not reported

Application Deadline: December 10

Prerequisite Coursework

Prerequisite coursework will be completed when students enter the program as college freshmen. All prerequisites must be completed with a grade "C" or better. There are no other prerequisites that must be completed prior to applying for matriculation.

No class statistics reported

PANCE Scores

5-year First Time Pass: 87%

Most Recent First Time Pass: 95%

Curriculum Structure

Didactic: 12 months (following completion of 62 credits of undergraduate prerequisite courses)

Clinical: 12 months

Rotations: 7 mandatory, 1 elective

Capstone Project: Required for graduation

Unique Program Features

Admissions Preference: First-year (freshman) students at Penn College will be offered conditionally reserved seats in the Physician Assistant major if they have a minimum ACT score at/or above 23 or SAT scores at/or above 550 in math, 500 in critical reading, and a writing sub-score of at least 8. These students must maintain both a Penn College graduation GPA and math/science GPA of 3.4, without any withdraw ("W"), "D," or "F" grades to retain their conditionally reserved seats in the major.

Class of 2017
Male: 42%
Female: 58%
Minority: 30.9%
GPA: 3.65
Science GPA: 3.63
GRE: Not required
Faculty to Student Ratio: Not reported
Average Healthcare Experience: Not reported

PANCE Scores
5-year First Time Pass: 97%

Most Recent First Time Pass: 98%

Curriculum Structure
Didactic: 14 months
Clinical: 12 months
Rotations: 7 mandatory (6 weeks long), 1 elective (4 weeks long)
Research Practicum: Required for graduation

PHILADELPHIA COLLEGE OF OSTEOPATHIC MEDICINE

Philadelphia College of Osteopathic Medicine
Email: PAadmissions@pcom.edu

Office of Admissions
4170 City Avenue
Philadelphia, PA 19131
Phone: 215-871-6772

Mission: The mission of the PCOM Physician Assistant Program is to educate highly qualified physician assistants, focusing on preparing them to become competent, compassionate, and comprehensive health care providers for clinical practice in the broad range of practice settings in both primary and specialty care fields that reflect the changing health care environment.

Accreditation: Continuing

Degree Offered: Master (MSPAS)

Start Date: June annually

Program Length: 26 months

Class Capacity: 57 students

Tuition: $86,663

GPA Requirement: Overall GPA 3.0; Science GPA 3.0;

Healthcare Experience: 200 hours required

PA Shadowing: Not required but recommended

Required Standardized Testing: None

Letters of Recommendation: Three required; One from a physician, PA, DO, or NP

Seat Deposit: $500

CASPA Participant: Yes

Supplemental Application: No

Admissions: Rolling

Application Deadline: December 1

Unique Program Features
Distant Campus: The PCOM PA program also has an approved distant campus in Suwanee, Georgia

Prerequisite Coursework
General Biology I and II with lab (2 semesters), Other Biology: Microbiology, Genetics, Cell Biology, etc. (1 semester)

Anatomy and Physiology with lab (2 semesters), General Chemistry I and II with lab (2 semesters), Other Chemistry: Organic Chemistry, Biochemistry (1 semester), Health-related Science course (Nutrition, Immunology, Virology) or Physics (1 semester), Social Sciences: Psychology, Sociology, Anthropology, etc. (3 semesters), Math (2 semesters)

PHILADELPHIA UNIVERSITY

Philadelphia University
Email:
paprogram
@philau.edu

4201 Henry Avenue
Philadelphia, PA 19144
Phone: 215-951-2908

No class statistics reported

PANCE Scores
5-year First Time Pass: 94%

Most Recent First Time Pass: 100%

Curriculum Structure
Didactic: 12 months
Clinical: 13 months
Rotations:
8 mandatory,
2 elective
(all 5 weeks long)
Capstone Project:
Not required

Mission: The mission of the Philadelphia University Physician Assistant Studies Program is to provide students with the foundation of knowledge, technical skills and critical thinking necessary to competently perform the functions of the physician assistant profession in an ethical, empathetic manner working with a licensed practicing physician. A secondary focus is to prepare students to provide comprehensive medical services to diverse under-served patient populations in inner-city and rural locations.

Accreditation:
Continuing

Degree Offered:
Master (MSPAS)

Start Date:
July annually

Program Length:
25 months

Class Capacity:
74 students

Tuition: $13,685
per trimester

GPA Requirement:
Overall GPA 3.25;
Science GPA 3.25

Healthcare Experience:
200 hours required

PA Shadowing:
Recommended but no specific number of hours required

Required Standardized Testing: Not required

Letters of Recommendation: Three required; One from a professor and one from a health care provider

Seat Deposit: $2,000

Unique Program Features

Two Campuses:
Philadelphia University now has two campuses for the Physician Assistant Studies program - one at Philadelphia University, East Falls, PA and one in Atlantic City, NJ.

Pre-PA Track: Available for interested high school seniors.

CASPA Participant: Yes

Supplemental Application: No

Admissions: Rolling

Application Deadline:
September 1

Prerequisite Coursework

Chemistry I and II with lab (2 semesters), Biology I and II with lab (2 semesters), Anatomy and Physiology I and II (2 semesters), Microbiology (1 semester), College Writing (1 semester), Statistics or Mathematics (1 semester), Introduction to Psychology (1 semester), Medical Terminology (1 course)

Class statistics

Faculty to Student Ratio: 1:41 (lectures); 1:13 (labs)

PANCE Scores

5-year First Time Pass: 96%

Most Recent First Time Pass: 97%

Curriculum Structure

Didactic: 15 months

Clinical: 12 months

Rotations: 8 mandatory (each 5 weeks long), 1 elective (6 weeks long)

Capstone Project: Not required

Unique Program Features

Direct Entry: Combined 5-year BS/MS option available.

SETON HILL UNIVERSITY

Seton Hill University
Email:
france@setonhill.edu

1 Seton Hill Drive
Greensburg, PA 15601
Phone: 724- 830-1097

Mission: The Physician Assistant Program at Seton Hill University is dedicated to the use of mobile technology to provide students with a quality academic and clinical education. All students will be trained as effective team members. Program emphasis is on delivering optimal care in an efficient, effective and professional manner.

Accreditation: Continuing

Degree Offered: Master (MSPA)

Start Date: January annually

Program Length: 27 months

Class Capacity: 41 students

Tuition: $91,910

GPA Requirement: Overall GPA 3.2; Science GPA 3.2; Prerequisite GPA 3.2

Healthcare Experience: 300 hours required

PA Shadowing: Required (12 hours total; 4 hours in three different medical or surgical specialties)

Required Standardized Testing: Not required

Letters of Recommendation: Three required; not from anyone specific

Seat Deposit: $450

CASPA Participant: Yes

Supplemental Application: No

Admissions: Not reported

Application Deadline: January 15

Prerequisite Coursework

Human Anatomy and Physiology I and II with lab (2 semesters), Chemistry I and II with lab (2 semesters), Organic Chemistry I and II with lab (2 semesters), Microbiology with lab (1 semester), Biochemistry (1 semester), Psychology (1 semester), Statistics (1 semester), Medical Terminology (1 course)

SALUS UNIVERSITY

Salus University

Email:
admissions@salus.edu

8360 Old York Road
Elkins Park, PA 19027
Phone: 215-780-1515

Mission: The mission of the Salus University Physician Assistant program is to graduate collaborative clinicians who will serve the health care needs of a worldwide community with intelligence, compassion, and integrity.

Accreditation:
Probation

Degree Offered:
Master (MMS)

Start Date:
August annually

Program Length:
25 months

Class Capacity:
50 students

Tuition: $71,810

GPA Requirement: Overall GPA 3.0; Science GPA 3.0

Healthcare Experience:
300 hours required

PA Shadowing: Required (20 hours)

Required Standardized Testing: GRE

Letters of Recommendation: Three required; One from a practicing physician assistant

Seat Deposit: $1,000

CASPA Participant: Yes

Supplemental Application: No

Admissions: Not reported

Application Deadline:
December 1

Class of 2017
Male: 36%
Female: 64%
Minority: 32%
GPA: 3.54
Science GPA:
Not reported
GRE: Not reported
Faculty to Student Ratio: Not reported
Average Healthcare Experience:
Not reported

PANCE Scores

5-year First Time Pass:
93%

Most Recent First Time Pass: 91%

Curriculum Structure

Didactic: 12 months

Clinical: 13 months

Rotations:
8 mandatory,
2 elective

Capstone Project:
Required for graduation

Prerequisite Coursework

Anatomy and Physiology I and II with lab (2 semesters), Biology I and II with lab (2 semesters), Chemistry I and II with lab (2 semesters), Microbiology, lab recommended but not required (1 semester), Organic Chemistry, lab recommended but not required (1 semester), Psychology (1 semester), Statistics or Biostatistics (1 semester), English Composition (1 semester), Medical Terminology (1 course)

Unique Program Features

Dual Degree: Salus offers a web-based Master of Public Health (MPH) degree program, Public Health Certificate Programs, and other initiatives that promote student engagement and impact, all with the ultimate goal of protecting and enhancing health and well being worldwide.

PANCE Scores

5-year First Time Pass: 96%

Most Recent First Time Pass: 100%

Curriculum Structure

Didactic: 12 months

Clinical: 12 months

Rotations:
8 mandatory,
1 elective
(all 5 weeks long)

Capstone Project: Not required

Prerequisite Coursework

Chemistry with lab (2 semesters), Human Anatomy and Physiology with lab (2 semesters), Microbiology with lab (1 semester), Psychology (1 semester)

Statistics or upper level Math (1 semester). All prerequisites must be completed with a grade "B" or better.

ST. FRANCIS UNIVERSITY

Saint Francis University
Email:
pa@francis.edu

Department of PA Sciences
117 Evergreen Drive
Loretto, PA 15940
Phone: 814-472-3130

Mission: To educate individuals as physician assistants to provide competent, compassionate and comprehensive health care to people and communities in need, as expressed through the Franciscan tradition.

Accreditation: Continuing

Degree Offered: Master (MPAS)

Start Date: May annually

Program Length: 24 months

Class Capacity: 55 students

Tuition: 93,050

CASPA Participant: Yes

Supplemental Application: No

Admissions: Rolling

Application Deadline: August 1

GPA Requirement:
Overall GPA 3.0;
Science GPA 3.0;
Prerequisite GPA 3.0

Healthcare Experience: 100 hours required

PA Shadowing: Required (40 of the 100 hours of required healthcare experience must be shadowing a PA)

Required Standardized Testing: Not required

Letters of Recommendation: Three required; not from anyone specific

Seat Deposit: $800

Unique Program Features

Direct Entry: 3+2 pre-PA track available for entering undergraduates.

Facilities: The DiSepio Institute for Rural Health and Wellness is a state-of-the-art 30,0000-square foot education and research center that is actively fulfilling its mission as a clinical training area for students as well as reaching out to underserved rural populations.

THOMAS JEFFERSON UNIVERSITY

Thomas Jefferson University
Email: jshpadmissions @jefferson.edu

130 S. 9th Street
Suite 100
Philadelphia, PA 19107
Phone: 215-503-8890

No class statistics reported

PANCE Scores
No scores available yet

Mission: The mission of the Thomas Jefferson University Department of Physician Assistant Studies is to use our model of interprofessional education to educate skilled, compassionate physician assistants prepared to provide leadership through our evolving healthcare system, dedicated to lifelong learning and service to the community.

Curriculum Structure
Didactic: 15 months
Clinical: 12 months
Rotations: 7 mandatory, 1 elective (all 5 weeks long)
Graduate Project: Required for graduation

Accreditation: Provisional

Degree Offered: Master (MSPAS)

Start Date: May annually

Program Length: 27 months

Class Capacity: 40 students

Tuition: $75,009

GPA Requirement: Overall GPA 3.0; Science GPA 3.0

Healthcare Experience: Preferred/Recommended

PA Shadowing: Recommended but no specific number of hours required

Required Standardized Testing: Not required

Letters of Recommendation: Three required; not from anyone specific

Seat Deposit: $300

Prerequisite Coursework

Biology with lab (2 semesters), Chemistry with lab (2 semesters), Anatomy with lab (1 semester), Physiology with lab (1 semester), Microbiology with lab (1 semester), Statistics (1 semester)

Psychology (1 semester)

CASPA Participant: Yes

Supplemental Application: Yes

Admissions: Rolling

Application Deadline: October 1

Unique Program Features

Facilities: A 66-seat, 1,605 square foot, state-of-the-art classroom and an additional 2,935 square foot laboratory space within the Dorrance Hamilton Building is dedicated for primary use by the PA program. Our PA students will have access to the Dr. Robert & Dorothy Rector Clinical Skills and Simulation Center (RCSSC) for clinical skills instruction and patient simulation.

Curriculum: One of the experiences that students participate in is our Health Mentors Program, an innovative longitudinal approach to teaching clinical medicine in multidisciplinary groups, pairing a patient living with chronic disease and an integrated group of students representing Sidney Kimmel Medical College and the Colleges of Pharmacy, Nursing and Health Professions. Through this experience, students learn how to better communicate with their colleagues and to appreciate the assets that each profession brings to the healthcare team.

Class of 2018

GPA: 3.55

Science GPA: 3.57

Average Healthcare Experience: 2,740 (and 60 hours of shadowing)

PANCE Scores

5-year First Time Pass: 94%

Most Recent First Time Pass: 97%

Curriculum Structure

Didactic: 12 months

Clinical: 12 months

Rotations: 8 mandatory, 1 elective (all 4 weeks long)

Capstone Project: Not required

Unique Program Features

None reported

CASPA Participant: Yes

Supplemental Application: No

UNIVERSITY OF PITTSBURGH

University of Pittsburgh
Email: admissions@shrs.pitt.edu

3010 William Pitt Way
Pittsburgh, PA 15238
Phone: 412-624-6743

Mission: mission of the Physician Assistant Program is to develop highly qualified physician assistants, who will serve as tomorrow's leaders in the provision of patient care, education and professional service. In order to achieve this mission, the PA Program has four main goals: To provide students with the required cognitive knowledge, affective behaviors, and psychomotor skills to consistently and reliably function as a physician assistant; To graduate skilled physician assistants who practice patient-centered care; To inspire a lifelong desire and responsibility for continued learning and advocacy within the health care profession; To inspire the graduates with motivation to pursue educational, research and administrative activities within the health care profession.

Accreditation: Continuing

Degree Offered: Master (MS)

Start Date: January annually

Program Length: 24 months

Class Capacity: 24 students

Tuition: $77,288 (in-state); $127,368 (out-of-state)

Admissions: Not reported

Application Deadline: November 1

GPA Requirement: Overall GPA 3.0; Science GPA 3.0; Prerequisite GPA 3.0

Healthcare Experience: 500 hours required

PA Shadowing: Recommended but no specific number of hours required

Required Standardized Testing: GRE

Letters of Recommendation: Three required; One from a professor, one from a supervisor of healthcare experience, and one character reference describing your commitment to leadership and service

Seat Deposit: $250

Prerequisite Coursework

Anatomy and Physiology with lab (2 semesters), Biology with lab (2 semesters), Chemistry with lab (2 semesters), English Composition/Writing (2 semesters), Microbiology with lab (1 semester), Organic Chemistry with lab (1 semester), Intro Psychology (1 semester), Upper level Psychology (1 semester), Statistics (1 semester), Medical Terminology (1 course)

UNIVERSITY OF THE SCIENCES OF PHILADELPHIA

University of the Sciences
Email: paprogram @usciences.edu

Box 27
600 South 43rd Street
Philadelphia, PA 19026
Phone: 215-596-7140

PANCE Scores
No scores available yet

Curriculum Structure
Didactic: 14 months
Clinical: 14 months
Rotations: 9 mandatory, 2 elective (all 5 weeks long)
Capstone Project: Required for graduation

Mission: The mission of the Graduate Professional Physician Assistant program is to provide a comprehensive curriculum that educates students to become providers of quality, evidence based medicine that encompasses the ethical, socioeconomic, and cultural sensitivities of each individual patient. The program will provide students with the motivation and skills to distinguish themselves as innovators and leaders in their field.

Accreditation: Provisional

Degree Offered: Master (MSPAS)Start Date: August annually

Program Length: 34 months

Class Capacity: 40 students

Tuition: $76,194

GPA Requirement: Overall GPA 3.2; Science GPA 3.2

Healthcare Experience: 400 hours required

PA Shadowing: Counts towards healthcare experience hours

Required Standardized Testing: Not required

Letters of Recommendation: Three required; not from anyone specific

Seat Deposit: $1,500

Unique Program Features
Schedule: Students get summers off from the program during didactic year.

CASPA Participant: Yes

Supplemental Application: Yes ($50 fee)

Admissions: Rolling

Application Deadline: November 1

Prerequisite Coursework
General Biology I and II with lab (2 semesters), Human Anatomy and Physiology (2 semesters), General Chemistry with lab (1 semester), Organic Chemistry or Biochemistry with lab (1 semester), Microbiology with lab (1 semester), Statistics (1 semester; note Business Statistics will not count), Psychology (1 semester)

RHODE ISLAND

BRYANT UNIVERSITY

Bryant University
Email:
pa_program@bryant.edu

1150 Douglas Pike
Smithfield, RI 02917
Phone: 401-232-6556

Mission: To improve universal access to health care by graduating highly competent and confident physician assistants prepared to provide exceptional quality, ethical patient-centered health care in a collaborative environment.

Accreditation:
Provisional

Degree Offered:
Master (MSPAS)

Start Date:
January annually

Program Length:
27 months

Class Capacity:
44 students

Tuition: $87,465

GPA Requirement:
Overall GPA 3.0;
Prerequisite GPA 3.0

Healthcare Experience:
2,000 hours required

PA Shadowing: Not reported

Required Standardized Testing: GRE

Letters of Recommendation: Three professional and one personal required

Seat Deposit: $800

CASPA Participant: Yes

Supplemental Application: Yes

Admissions: Not reported

Application Deadline:
October 1

Prerequisite Coursework

Biology with lab, Chemistry with lab, Human Anatomy and Physiology, Microbiology, Biochemistry or Organic Chemistry with lab, Psychology, Statistics

All prerequisites must be completed with a grade of "C" or better. All prerequisites must be completed by September 1.

No class statistics reported

PANCE Scores

5-year First Time Pass: Not yet available

Most Recent First Time Pass: Not yet available

Curriculum Structure

Didactic: 12 months

Clinical: 15 months

Rotations:
10 mandatory,
1 elective,
1 mini rotation
(all 4 weeks long)

Capstone Project: No project requirement

Unique Program Features

Didactics: The human anatomy course takes place at Brown University's medical education building.

Facilities: All new, high-tech classrooms and laboratories, including a high-fidelity simulation lab and a physical exam lab.

Class of 2017

Male: 25%

Female: 75%

GPA: 3.62

Science GPA: 3.59

GRE: Verbal – 60%;
Quantitative – 57%;
Analytical – 64%

Faculty to Student Ratio: 1:10.4

Average Healthcare Experience: 3,000 hours

PANCE Scores

Not available yet

Curriculum Structure

Didactic: 12 months

Clinical: 12 months

Rotations: 7 mandatory, 2 elective (each 5 weeks)

CapstoneProject: Required for graduation

Prerequisite Coursework

Anatomy and Physiology with labs, Biology with labs, Chemistry (Organic and Biochemistry preferred) with labs, Math (Statistics preferred), English, Psychology/Sociology/ Behavioral Science

JOHNSON AND WALES

Johnson & Wales University
Email:
Katie.Spolidoro@jwu.edu

8 Abbott Park Place
Providence, RI 2903
Phone: 401-598-4558

Mission: The mission of the Physician Assistant Studies program at JWU is to educate students to become collaborative practitioners with the respect, empathy and trust inherent to patient-centered, humanistic health care. Maintaining a relationship of trust and caring is central to becoming a health care professional, whether your goal is to stay in Rhode Island to care for Rhode Islanders, or go where a growing career opportunity takes you.

Accreditation: Provisional

Degree Offered: Master (MSPAS)

Start Date: June annually

Program Length: 24 months

Class Capacity: 24 students

Tuition: $87,984

GPA Requirement: Overall GPA 3.0; Science GPA 3.0

Healthcare Experience: 250 hours

PA Shadowing: Required— Shadowing of PAs in more than one practice type is preferred

Required Standardized Testing: GRE

Letters of Recommendation: Three required; not from anyone specific

Seat Deposit: $1,000

CASPA Participant: Yes

Supplemental Application: No

Admissions: Rolling

Application Deadline: March 1

Unique Program Features

Admissions Preference: Articulation agreements are in place with local colleges and universities, with the goal of recruiting students who desire to practice in Rhode Island upon completion of their training.

Facilities: Brand new, state-of-the-art facility built specifically for the PA program. The facility is set up to maximize information sharing, teamwork and collaboration between students, faculty and community colleagues, with (1) Lecture halls with global teleconferencing capabilities, (2) "Active learning" classrooms that can be easily reconfigured for group work or lectures, depending on the need, (3) Cadaver-based anatomy lab with access to e-study guides at each dissection station and a (4) Clinical practice center similar to a hospital emergency room.

SOUTH CAROLINA

MEDICAL UNIVERSITY OF SOUTH CAROLINA

Medical University of
South Carolina
Email:
chpstusv@musc.edu

Education and Student Life
171 Ashley Avenue
Charleston, SC 29425
Phone: 843-792-1913

Mission: To educate highly competent physician assistants who are compassionate, culturally aware, and attuned to the primary care needs of the people of SC and beyond. They will be prepared to provide quality, state-of-the-art, patient-centered care as integral members of physician-led health care teams; contribute to the dissemination of new knowledge to improve physician assistant education and health care; advocate for the physician assistant profession; and help meet the health needs of larger community through education and service.

Accreditation:
Continuing

Degree Offered:
Master (MSPAS)

Start Date:
May annually

Program Length:
27 months

Class Capacity:
60 students

Tuition:
In-state: $59,653;
Out-of-state: $87,261

GPA Requirement: Overall GPA 3.0; Science GPA 3.0 Prerequisite GPA 3.0

Healthcare Experience:
Recommended

PA Shadowing: Not required

Required Standardized Testing: GRE

Letters of Recommendation: Three required; minimum of one from a physician, PA, or NP

Seat Deposit: $1,000

CASPA Participant: No

Supplemental Application: Yes

Admissions: Non-rolling

Application Deadline:
September 15

Prerequisite Coursework

Mathematics (3 credits), Statistics or Biostatistics (3 credits), General Chemistry with lab (8 credits), Organic or Biochemistry (3 credits), Biology with lab (4 credits), Anatomy with lab (4 credits), Physiology with lab (4 credits), Microbiology with lab (4 credits), Medical Terminology (1 credit), Behavioral Sciences (General Psychology + six credits of psychology electives or sociology), Humanities (12 credits), English (6 credits), Electives (30 credits). Prerequisite math, science, and behavioral sciences must be completed in the last 10 years.

Class of 2017
Male: 23%
Female: 77%
Minority: 7%
GPA: 3.79
Science GPA: 3.89
GRE: not reported
Faculty to Student Ratio: not reported
Average Healthcare Experience:
500 hours

PANCE Scores
5-year First Time Pass: 96%

Most Recent First Time Pass: 100%

Curriculum Structure
Didactic: 15 months
Clinical: 12 months
Rotations:
7 mandatory, 1 primary care elective, 1 elective, unspecified duration

Unique Program Features
Admissions Preference: Approximately 50% of each class is made up of South Carolina residents, while the other 50% comes from other states.

SOUTH DAKOTA

UNIVERSITY OF SOUTH DAKOTA

The University of South Dakota
Email: pa@usd.edu

PA Program, 414 East Clark Street
Vermillion, SD 57069
Phone: 605-677-5128

PANCE Scores

5-year First Time Pass: 92%

Most Recent First Time Pass: 92%

Curriculum Structure

Didactic: 12 months

Clinical: 12 months

Rotations: 8 mandatory, 2 electives;

Master's Project: Required for graduation

Mission: The Physician Assistant Studies Program at the University of South Dakota provides a comprehensive primary care education that prepares graduates to deliver high quality healthcare to meet the needs of patients in South Dakota and the region.

Accreditation: Continued

Degree Offered: Master (MSPAS)

Start Date: July annually

Program Length: 24 months

Class Capacity: 25 students

Tuition: In-state: $22,812; Out-of-state: $66,524

GPA Requirement: Overall GPA 3.0; Prerequisite GPA 3.0

Healthcare Experience: Preferred, not required

PA Shadowing: Preferred, not required

Required Standardized Testing: Not required

Letters of Recommendation: Two required; no one specific

Seat Deposit: $650

CASPA Participant: Yes

Supplemental Application: Yes

Admissions: Not specified

Application Deadline: September 1

Prerequisite Coursework

Biology (8 credits), Chemistry with lab (8 credits), Anatomy and Physiology with lab (8 credits), Microbiology with lab (4 credits), Biochemistry (3 credits), General Psychology (3 credits), Abnormal Psychology (3 credits), Statistics (2 credits). Courses are recommended to be completed in the last 10 years and can be in progress at the time of application

Unique Program Features

Admissions Preference: The admissions committee gives preference to applicants with an overall and prerequisite GPA of 3.20 or greater, desire for practice in primary care or medically underserved area, direct patient contact of 1,000 hours or greater, those with strong ties to South Dakota (resident, one or both parents are residents, graduated from high school in South Dakota, graduated from an accredited South Dakota University or College). The program accepts non-resident students and encourages them to apply.

TENNESSEE

BETHEL UNIVERSITY

Bethel University
Email:
paprogram@bethelu.edu

302B Tyson Avenue
Paris, TN 38242
Phone: 731-407-7650

Mission: The Bethel University mission is to create opportunities for members of the learning community to develop to their highest potential as whole persons-intellectually, spiritually, socially, and physically, in a Christian environment. It is the Physician Assistant Program's mission to create opportunities for the members of the learning community interested in healthcare to ultimately graduate as competent, caring healthcare professionals who practice medicine within an ethical framework grounded in Christian principles.

Accreditation:
Continued

Degree Offered:
Master (MSPAS)

Start Date:
January annually

Program Length:
27 months

Class Capacity:
50 students

Tuition: $80,500

GPA Requirement: No minimum

Healthcare Experience:
Recommended

PA Shadowing:
40 hours required

Required Standardized Testing: GRE

Letters of Recommendation: Three required; one from a MD, DO, PA, or NP; one from a MD, DO, PA, or NP; one from a supervisor or advisor/professor

Seat Deposit: $1,000

CASPA Participant: Yes

Supplemental Application: Yes

Admissions: Rolling

Application Deadline:
October 1

Class of 2017
Male: 42%
Female: 58%
Minority:
not reported
GPA: 3.36
Science GPA:
not reported
GRE Quantitative:
153
GRE Verbal: 154
GRE Analytical: 4.1
Faculty to Student Ratio: not reported
Average Healthcare Experience:
3,567 hours
Average Shadowing Hours: 194 hours

PANCE Scores
5-year First Time Pass:
96%

Most Recent First Time Pass: 95%

Curriculum Structure
Didactic: 12 months
Clinical: 15 months
Rotations:
8 mandatory,
3 elective,
5 weeks each

Prerequisite Coursework

General Biology I and II, General Chemistry I and II, Human Anatomy and Physiology I and II, Microbiology or Bacteriology, Psychology, Human Genetics. No prerequisites older than 5 years will be accepted, unless you have been employed full time in the health care field since completion of those prerequisites.

Unique Program Features

Business of Medicine: This course is taken during clinical year and educates students on group practice models, management, human resources, insurance products, CPT and ICD coding, third party reimbursement as well as the potential impact of health care reform.

Medical Mission Trip: Over Spring Break in March of 2015 thirteen students, faculty, and staff members from Bethel's College of Health Sciences traveled to southern Belize to set up medical clinics and administer medical care.

Community Service: The students participate in several volunteer commitments throughout the year including volunteering at a free clinic, toy drives, and 5k runs.

PANCE Scores

5-year First Time Pass: 69% (only one class has graduated)

Most Recent First Time Pass: 69%

Curriculum Structure

Didactic: 15 months

Clinical: 12 months

Rotations: 9 mandatory, 2 elective, 4 weeks each

CHRISTIAN BROTHERS UNIVERSITY

Christian Brothers University
Email: pas@cbu.edu

650 East Parkway South
Memphis, TN 38104
Phone: 901-321-3388

Mission: The mission of the Physician Assistant Studies program at CBU is to meet the needs of those suffering from a lack of quality primary care services by training healthcare providers who deliver excellent and compassionate care using current evidence-based medical information and knowledge. Our diverse graduates become life-long learners collaborating with physicians and other healthcare workers in their communities to advance the profession of the Physician Assistant.

Unique Program Features

Applications: The program is not accepting new applications at this time. They are reapplying for Accreditation – Provisional Status and voluntarily withdrawing from ARC-PA accreditation in May 2017.

Accreditation: Probation

Degree Offered: Master (MSPAS)

Start Date: January annually

Program Length: 27 months

Class Capacity: 42 students

Tuition: $76,420

GPA Requirement: Overall GPA 2.8; Science GPA 2.8; Prerequisite GPA 2.8

Healthcare Experience: Recommended

PA Shadowing: Not required

Required Standardized Testing: GRE

Letters of Recommendation: Three required; all three letters must be from a health care professional

Seat Deposit: $1,130

CASPA Participant: No

Supplemental Application: No

Admissions: Not specified

Application Deadline: July 1

Prerequisite Coursework

Anatomy with lab (4 credits), Physiology with lab (4 credits), General Chemistry with lab (8 credits), General Biology with lab (8 credits), Genetics with lab (4 credits), Organic Chemistry or Biochemistry with lab (4 credits), Microbiology with lab (4 credits), General Psychology (3 credits), Medical Terminology, English Composition (6 credits), College Algebra or higher (3 credits).

LINCOLN MEMORIAL UNIVERSITY

Lincoln Memorial
Email:
paadmissions
@lmunet.edu

6965 Cumberland Gap Parkway
Harrogate, TN 37752
Phone: Not provided

Mission: The Physician Assistant Program at Lincoln Memorial University-DeBusk College of Osteopathic Medicine recruits, educates and mentors a diverse group of students to become physician assistants providing quality health care. It emphasizes primary care and preventive medicine and seeks to interest students in providing care to the medically underserved population within the Appalachian Region and beyond; uses didactic and clinical training and promotes physician/PA team care; fosters an appreciation for research, leadership and flexibility in meeting the changing needs of the health care climate; empowers faculty and students to be advocates for the physician assistant profession for the delivery of primary health care.

Accreditation:
Continuing
Degree Offered:
Master (MMS)
Start Date:
May annually
Program Length:
27 months
Class Capacity:
96 students
Tuition: $83,650

CASPA Participant:
Yes

Supplemental Application: Yes

Admissions: Rolling

Application Deadline: November 1

GPA Requirement:
Overall GPA 2.75;
Science GPA 2.75;

Healthcare Experience:
150 hours required

PA Shadowing: 40 hours required, 20 of which must be in primary care

Required Standardized Testing: GRE

Letters of Recommendation: Three required; one letter must be from a PA, one from a PA, physician, dentist, podiatrist, or optometrist, and one must be from an academic advisor, science/math professor, or current/recent employer.

Seat Deposit: $500

Prerequisite Coursework

General Biology I and II with lab (8 credits), Human Anatomy with lab, Human Physiology, General Chemistry I and II with lab (8 credits), Organic Chemistry I and II with lab (7 credits), Biochemistry (3 credits), General Psychology (3 credits), Psychology Elective (3 credits), Microbiology with lab (4 credits), English (6 credits), Mathematics (3 credits), Medical Terminology, Statistics (2 credits).

PANCE Scores

5-year First Time Pass: 94%

Most Recent First Time Pass: 97%

Curriculum Structure

Didactic: 15 months

Clinical: 12 months

Rotations: 7 mandatory, 1 elective, 6 weeks each

Capstone Research Project: required to graduate

Prerequisite Coursework

Anatomy and Physiology I and II with labs (8 credits), General Chemistry I and II with labs (8 credits), Biology I and II with labs (8 credits), English (6 credits), Statistics or Algebra or Calculus or Finite Math (6 credits), Humanities or Social Science (6 credits).

SOUTH COLLEGE

South College
Email:
pa_program
@southcollegetn.edu

400 Goody's Lane
Parkside Campus
Knoxville, TN 37922
Phone: 865-251-1800

Mission: The Mission of the Masters of Health Science Physician Assistant Studies Program is to educate highly qualified physician assistants, preparing them to become competent, compassionate, and comprehensive health care providers for clinical practice in rural and urban areas, focusing on underserved communities.

Accreditation: Continuing

Degree Offered: Master (MHS)

Start Date: October annually

Program Length: 27 months

Class Capacity: 85 students

Tuition: $81,900

GPA Requirement: Overall GPA 2.75; Science GPA 2.75; Prerequisite GPA 2.75

Healthcare Experience: Recommended

PA Shadowing: Not required

Required Standardized Testing: GRE

Letters of Recommendation: Three required; one from a physician, PA or NP

Seat Deposit: $1,500

CASPA Participant: Yes

Supplemental Application: Yes

Admissions: Not specified

Application Deadline: March 1

Unique Program Features

Simulation: Throughout the curriculum the program uses high fidelity simulation exercises focusing on developing PA competencies for practice.

VET-UP: This program is specifically designed for medics and corpsmen candidates as a bridging program to enter the Physician Assistant Program at South College. Candidates must have 4 years military service as a medic or corpsmen and be in the process of completing a BS degree with a focus on health sciences.

TREVECCA NAZARENE UNIVERSITY

Trevecca Nazarene University
Email: moverstreet@trevecca.edu

333 Murfreesboro Road
Nashville, TN 37210
Phone: 615-248-1225

Mission: The Physician Assistant program exists to prepare professionally competent physician assistants who will use their skills to serve their communities in compassionate ministry.

Accreditation: Continuing

Degree Offered: Master (MSM)

Start Date: May annually

Program Length: 27 months

Class Capacity: 50 students

Tuition: $92,300

GPA Requirement: Overall GPA 3.25; Science GPA 3.25;

Healthcare Experience: 250 hours required

PA Shadowing: 40 hours required

Required Standardized Testing: GRE

Letters of Recommendation: Three required; one from a PA

Seat Deposit: $1,000

CASPA Participant: Yes

Supplemental Application: No

Admissions: Not specified

Application Deadline: October 1

Class of 2017

Male: not reported
Female: not reported
Minority: not reported
GPA: 3.72
Science GPA 3.66
GRE Combined: 310
Faculty to Student Ratio: not reported
Average Healthcare Experience: not reported

PANCE Scores

5-year First Time Pass: 94%

Most Recent First Time Pass: 98%

Curriculum Structure

Didactic: 15 months
Clinical: 12 months
Rotations: 7 mandatory, 1 elective, 6 weeks each

Prerequisite Coursework

Human Anatomy and Physiology with lab (8 credits), General Chemistry I and II with lab (8 credits), General Psychology (3 credits), Microbiology with lab (4 credits), Developmental Psychology (3 credits), Medical Terminology (1 credit or certificate). All courses must be taken within 7 years of matriculation.

Unique Program Features

Medical Mission Trips: Students can participate in rotations and trips to Zambia, Papua New Guinea, and Haiti.

Early Clinical Exposure: PA students participate in learning experiences with The Clinic at Mercury Courts and Room In The Inn which serve Nashville's medically underserved and homeless population throughout the didactic phase of the program.

PANCE Scores

5-year First Time Pass: 92% (only one class has graduated)

Most Recent First Time Pass: 92%

Curriculum Structure

Didactic: 12 months

Clinical: 12 months

Rotations: 9 mandatory, 2 elective, 4 weeks each

Capstone: required for graduation

Unique Program Features

Academic Medical Center: This is the only program in TN that boasts being part of an academic medical center and providing students with access to the resources therein.

UNIVERSITY OF TENNESSEE HEALTH SCIENCE CENTER

University of Tennessee Health Science Center
Email: paprogram@uthsc.edu

910 Madison Avenue
Suite 520
Memphis, TN 38163
Phone: 901-448-8000

Mission: The mission of the University of Tennessee Health Science Center's Physician Assistant program is to prepare a diverse group of highly skilled Physician Assistant practitioners who are dedicated to improving access and providing high quality primary and/or specialty health care as part of interprofessional teams and who are committed to lifelong learning and to increasing the knowledge base of the profession.

Accreditation: Provisional

Degree Offered: Master (MMS)

Start Date: January annually

Program Length: 24 months

Class Capacity: 30 students

Tuition:
In-state: $43,680;
Out-of-state: $74,880

GPA Requirement: Overall GPA 3.2

Healthcare Experience: 500 hours required

PA Shadowing: Recommended

Required Standardized Testing: GRE

Letters of Recommendation: Two required; no one specific

Seat Deposit: $1,000

CASPA Participant: Yes

Supplemental Application: No

Admissions: Not specified

Application Deadline: November 1

Prerequisite Coursework

Anatomy and Physiology with lab (8 credits), Biology with lab (8 credits), Microbiology (3 credits), Chemistry with lab (8 credits), Medical Terminology (1 credit), General Psychology or Sociology or Anthropology (3 credits), Math (3 credits).

TEXAS

BAYLOR COLLEGE OF MEDICINE

Baylor College of
Medicine
Email:
paprogram@bcm.edu

One Baylor Plaza
M108
Houston, TX 77030
Phone: not provided

Class of 2017
Male: not reported
Female: not reported
Minority:
not reported
GPA: 3.63
Science GPA:
not reported
GRE Total: 317
GRE Analytical: 4.4
*Faculty to Student
Ratio:* not reported
*Average Healthcare
Experience:*
not reported

PANCE Scores
5-year First Time Pass:
97%
Most Recent First Time
Pass: 98%

Curriculum Structure
Didactic: 13 months
Clinical: 17 months
Rotations:
11 mandatory,
0 elective,
4-8 weeks each
*Master's Research
Paper:* required for
graduation

Mission: The intent of the PA Program is to produce future generations of PAs for leadership roles in clinical practice settings where physicians direct care, in the health policy arena with other disciplines, as managers of healthcare delivery organizations and facilities, as faculty members within academic institutions educating future PAs, and as providers engaged in the transfer of best evidence to the clinical environment.

Accreditation:
Continuing
Degree Offered:
Master (MSPA)
Start Date:
June annually
Program Length:
30 months
Class Capacity:
40 students
Tuition: $46,340

CASPA Participant:
Yes
**Supplemental
Application:** Yes
Admissions: Not
specified
**Application
Deadline:** September 1

GPA Requirement:
Overall GPA 3.0;
Science GPA 3.0
Healthcare Experience:
500 hours required
PA Shadowing:
Recommended
**Required Standardized
Testing:** GRE (minimum 153
on verbal, 144 on quantitative,
and 3.5 on analytical)
**Letters of
Recommendation:** Three
required; no one specific
Seat Deposit: $300

Prerequisite Coursework

Human Anatomy with lab (4 credits), Human Physiology with lab (4 credits), Microbiology with lab (4 credits), General Chemistry with lab (8 credits), Organic Chemistry with lab (4 credits), Statistics (3 credits), General Psychology (3 credits), Psychology Elective (3 credits), English Expository Writing (3 credits)

Unique Program Features

Texas Medical Center: As the largest medical center in the world it offers world class facilities for the training of fellows, residents, medical, psychology, pharmacy, nursing, and social work students and others in the allied health disciplines.

Multicultural Experiences: A mix of public and private institutions and community-based facilities provides a rich exposure to patients and families from many cultures and ethnic groups that expose students to health beliefs and practices influenced by cultural origins that provide an understanding of how to approach the provision of patient-centered care.

Interdisciplinary Education: Team-based instruction occurs within the didactic and clinical phases of the curriculum with experiences involving various mixes of medical, nurse anesthesia, physician assistant, pharmacy, social work, and nursing students ensuring a rich experience in the area of role socialization.

INTERSERVICE

Interservice PA Program
Email: maria.r.charles.civ @mail.mil

3599 Winfield Scott Road
Academy of Health Sciences, Graduate School
JBSA Fort Sam Houston, TX 78234-6130
Phone: 210-221-6776

Mission: To provide the uniformed services with highly competent, compassionate physician assistants who model integrity, strive for leadership excellence, and are committed to lifelong learning.

PANCE Scores

5-year First Time Pass: 97%

Most Recent First Time Pass: 100%

Curriculum Structure

Didactic: 16 months

Clinical: 13 months

Rotations: 11 mandatory, 1 elective, variable duration

Master's Research Paper: required for graduation

Prerequisite Coursework

A minimum of 60 semester hours with emphasis in science course work. SAT, Basic Life Support, Service Unique Applicant Package.

Accreditation: Continuing

Degree Offered: Master (MSPA)

Start Date: August annually

Program Length: 29 months

Class Capacity: 80 students

Tuition: $0

GPA Requirement: Overall GPA 2.75; Science GPA 2.8; Prerequisite GPA 2.75

Healthcare Experience: Recommended

PA Shadowing: Not required

Required Standardized Testing: None

Letters of Recommendation: One required from a military PA

Seat Deposit: None

CASPA Participant: No

Supplemental Application: No

Admissions: Not specified

Application Deadline: None

Unique Program Features

Applicants: This program is only for Service members of the Army, Navy, Air Force, Coast Guard, Army Reserves, and Army National Guard. Marine Corps applicants also encouraged - apply with Navy.

Rotations: Applicants are assigned to a single core site where they complete the majority of their rotations.

TEXAS TECH UNIVERSITY HEALTH SCIENCES CENTER

Texas Tech University
Health Sciences Center
Email:
allied.health
@ttuhsc.edu

3601 4th Street
MS 6294
Lubbock, TX 79430
Phone: 806-743-3220

Mission: The mission of the Texas Tech University Health Sciences Center Physician Assistant Program is to offer the primary care physician assistant student the finest medical education in the best learning environment available and to uphold the TTUHSC mission of educating quality medical professionals to provide compassionate health care to the underserved regions of West Texas and beyond.

Accreditation:
Probation

Degree Offered:
Master (MPAS)

Start Date:
May annually

Program Length:
27 months

Class Capacity:
60 students

Tuition:
In-state: $29,862;
Out-of-state: $79,002

GPA Requirement:
Overall GPA 3.0;
Science GPA 3.0;
Prerequisite GPA 3.0

Healthcare Experience:
Not required

PA Shadowing:
Recommended, not required

Required Standardized Testing: GRE

Letters of Recommendation: Three required; no one specific

Seat Deposit: $100

CASPA Participant: Yes

Supplemental Application: Yes

Admissions: Rolling

Application Deadline:
December 1

Class of 2017

Male: not reported
Female: not reported
Minority: 11%
GPA: 3.56
Science GPA: 3.43
GRE Quantitative: 43rd percentile
GRE Verbal: 45th percentile
GRE Analytical: 42nd percentile
Faculty to Student Ratio: not reported
Average Healthcare Experience: not reported

PANCE Scores

5-year First Time Pass: 95%

Most Recent First Time Pass: 95%

Curriculum Structure

Didactic: 15 months
Clinical: 12 months
Rotations:
7 mandatory, 1 selective, 6 weeks duration
Master's Project:
required for graduation

Prerequisite Coursework

Genetics (3 credits), Microbiology (4 credits), Human Anatomy and Physiology (8 credits), Organic Chemistry or Biochemistry (4 credits), Psychology (3 credits), Statistics (3 credits). No more than 9 credits can be in progress at the time of application.

Unique Program Features

Rotations: Applicants are assigned to a single region where they complete the majority of their clinical rotations. No region is limited to one city however. Example regions include El Paso, Lubbock, Amarillo, Abilene, and Odessa/Midland.

Class of 2018

Male: not reported

Female: not reported

Minority: not reported

GPA: 3.71

Science GPA: 3.67

GRE Combined: 58th percentile

Faculty to Student Ratio: not reported

Average Healthcare Experience: not reported

PANCE Scores

5-year First Time Pass: 99%

Most Recent First Time Pass: 100%

Curriculum Structure

Didactic: 18 months

Clinical: 16 months

Rotations: 10 mandatory, 1 elective, 4-8 weeks each

UNIVERSITY OF NORTH TEXAS HEALTH SCIENCES CENTER FORT WORTH

UNT Health Science Center
UNT Admissions

3500 Camp Bowie Boulevard
Fort Worth, TX 76107
Phone: 817-735-2003
Email: paadmissions@unthsc.edu

Mission: To create solutions for a healthier community by preparing graduates with knowledge and skills needed for physician assistant practice, emphasizing primary care medicine and meeting the healthcare needs of underserved populations

Accreditation: Continuing

Degree Offered: Master (MPAS)

Start Date: July annually

Program Length: 34 months

Class Capacity: 75 students

Tuition:
In-state: $23,398;
Out-of-state: $82,298

GPA Requirement: Overall GPA 2.85

Healthcare Experience: Recommended

PA Shadowing: Recommended

Required Standardized Testing: GRE

Letters of Recommendation: Two required; no one specific

Seat Deposit: None

CASPA Participant: Yes

Supplemental Application: No

Admissions: Rolling

Application Deadline: November 1

Unique Program Features

Early Clinical Exposure: Students complete supervised clinical experiences throughout the didactic portion of the curriculum to begin to integrate classroom knowledge with clinical knowledge.

Underserved Rotation: Every student completes a rotation dedicated to working with an underserved population.

Prerequisite Coursework

General or Introductory Psychology (3 credits), Behavior/Social Science Elective (3 credits), College Algebra or higher (3 credits), Statistics (3 credits), Anatomy with lab (4 credits), Physiology with lab (4 credits), Organic Chemistry with lab (4 credits), Microbiology (4 credits), Genetics or Immunology or Cell Biology or Biochemistry or Neuroscience or Pharmacology or Histology (6 credits). Courses must be completed prior to December 31 of application year.

UNIVERSITY OF TEXAS HEALTH SCIENCE CENTER AT SAN ANTONIO

University of Texas HS Center at San Antonio
Email: pastudies @uthscsa.edu

Department of Physician Assistant Studies
7703 Floyd Curl Drive, MC 6249
San Antonio, TX 78229
Phone: 210-567-4240

Mission: The mission of The University of Texas Health Science Center at San Antonio, Department of Physician Assistant Studies is to prepare primary health care providers who will contribute to the improvement of the mental, social, and physical well-being of the underserved and vulnerable people of South Texas. This mission will be accomplished through culturally appropriate, socially relevant education, service, and scholarship.

Accreditation:
Continuing

Degree Offered:
Master (MPAS)

Start Date:
May annually

Program Length:
30 months

Class Capacity:
45 students

Tuition:
In-state: $34,905;
Out-of-state: $73,615

GPA Requirement:
Overall GPA 3.0;
Science GPA 3.0

Healthcare Experience:
500 hours required

PA Shadowing:
100 hours required

Required Standardized Testing: GRE

Letters of Recommendation: Two required; no one specific

Seat Deposit: $250

CASPA Participant: Yes

Supplemental Application: Yes

Admissions: Not specified

Application Deadline:
September 1

Prerequisite Coursework

Biology I and II with lab (8 credits), Human Anatomy with lab (4 credits), Human Physiology (3 credits), Organic Chemistry I and II with lab (8 credits), Biochemistry (3 credits), Microbiology (3 credits), Genetics (3 credits), Psychology (3 credits), Statistics (3 credits). All must be completed by application deadline.

No class statistics reported

PANCE Scores
5-year First Time Pass: 94%

Most Recent First Time Pass: 100%

Curriculum Structure
Didactic: 15 months

Clinical: 15 months

Rotations:
8 mandatory, 2 elective, 1 selective, 4 weeks each; One 4 month career-focused rotation

Quality Improvement Project: required for graduation

Unique Program Features

Career-Focused Rotation: Students choose a rotation of interest that they spend 4 months completing. They develop advanced skills and knowledge in an area of interest to prepare them for future employment.

Primary Care Focus: The program is committed to primary care with students completing 3 primary care rotations and the program fostering graduate employment in South Texas in underserved areas and populations.

UNIVERSITY OF TEXAS MEDICAL BRANCH AT GALVESTON

University of Texas - Medical Branch and Galveston

301 University Boulevard
Galveston, TX 77555-1145
Phone: 409-772-3048
Email: pasadmis@utmb.edu

Mission: Prepare and graduate an academically and clinically exceptional physician assistants.

Accreditation: Continuing

Degree Offered: Master (MPAS)

Start Date: July annually

Program Length: 26 months

Class Capacity: 90 students

Tuition:
In-state: $29,700;
Out-of-state: $70,300

GPA Requirement:
Overall GPA 3.0;
Science GPA 3.0

Healthcare Experience: Recommended

PA Shadowing: Not required

Required Standardized Testing: GRE

Letters of Recommendation: Three required; no one specific

Seat Deposit: $200

CASPA Participant: Yes

Supplemental Application: Yes

Admissions: Not specified

Application Deadline: September 1

Unique Program Features

Tradition: The program has a 42 year history of PA education, still teaches anatomy with a cadaver lab, and has an emphasis on educating culturally competent PAs.

Rotations: International rotations are available as well as rotations within UTMB, VA clinics, Shriner's Burn Hospital, MD Anderson Cancer Hospital, and other outpatient rural and underserved settings.

Prerequisite Coursework

Biological Sciences with lab (8 credits), Microbiology or Bacteriology (3-4 credits), Immunology or Virology (3 credits), Genetics (3 credits), Anatomy with lab (4 credits), Physiology with lab (4 credits), Chemistry with lab (8 credits), Organic Chemistry or Biochemistry (304 credits), Behavioral Sciences (6 credits), Statistics (3 credits), College Algebra or higher (3 credits).

UNIVERSITY OF TEXAS RIO GRANDE VALLEY

University of Texas Pan American
Email:
pad@utpa.edu

1201 West University Drive
Edinburg, TX 78539
Phone: 956-665-7049

Mission: The mission of the Physician Assistant Studies Department (PAD) at the University of Texas - Pan American (UTPA) is to provide an advanced education to physician assistant students who are capable of rendering preventive and primary health care to the multicultural population of South Texas.

Accreditation:
Continuing

Degree Offered:
Master (MPAS)

Start Date:
August annually

Program Length:
28 months

Class Capacity:
50 students

Tuition:
In-state: $25,430;
Out-of-state: $60,590

GPA Requirement:
Overall GPA 3.0;
Science GPA 3.0

Healthcare Experience:
Recommended

PA Shadowing: Not required

Required Standardized Testing: None

Letters of Recommendation: Three required; no one specific

Seat Deposit: $200

CASPA Participant: Yes

Supplemental Application: Yes

Admissions: Not rolling

Application Deadline:
October 1

Class of 2016
Male: 31%
Female: 69%
Minority: 62%
GPA: 3.50
Science GPA: 3.45
GRE: not required
Faculty to Student Ratio: not reported
Average Healthcare Experience:
not reported

PANCE Scores
5-year First Time Pass:
77%

Most Recent First Time
Pass: 90%

Curriculum Structure
Didactic: 14 months
Clinical: 12 months
Rotations:
8 mandatory,
1 elective,
4 weeks each
Master's Capstone:
required for
graduation

Prerequisite Coursework

General Biology I and II (6 credits), Genetics (3 credits), Microbiology (3 credits), Anatomy and Physiology I and II (6 credits), General Chemistry I and II (6 credits), Organic Chemistry or Biochemistry (3 credits), Statistics (3 credits), Introductory Psychology or Abnormal Psychology (3 credits).

Unique Program Features

Diversity: The program typically accepts >50% of its class as minority students

Spanish Language: Fluency or experience with the Spanish language is desirable given the location of the program in an area of dense Spanish speakers.

PANCE Scores

5-year First Time Pass: 100%

Most Recent First Time Pass: 100%

Curriculum Structure

Didactic: 15 months

Clinical: 15 months

Rotations:
8 mandatory,
1 selective, 1 elective
4-8 weeks each

Prerequisite Coursework

Human Anatomy with lab (4 credits), Human Physiology with lab (4 credits), Genetics (3 credits), Psychology (3 credits), General Chemistry with lab (8 credits), Organic Chemistry with lab (4 credits), Microbiology with lab (4 credits), College Algebra or higher (3 credits). All courses must have been completed in the last 10 years and must be completed by December 31 in the year you apply.

UNIVERSITY OF TEXAS SOUTHWESTERN

UT Southwestern
Email:
PA.SSHP
@UTSouthwestern.edu

5323 Harry Hines Boulevard
Suite V4.114
Dallas, TX 75390-9090
Phone: 214-648-1701

Mission: To excel in the art and science of physician assistant education. To encourage leadership, service, and excellence among our faculty, staff, students and graduates. To promote primary health care delivery to a diverse and dynamic population. To foster a commitment to evidence-based lifelong learning.

Accreditation: Continuing

Degree Offered: Master (MPAS)

Start Date: May annually

Program Length: 30 months

Class Capacity: 42 students

Tuition:
In-state: $29,572;
Out-of-state: $70,116

GPA Requirement:
Overall GPA 3.0;
Science GPA 3.0;
Prerequisite 2.0

Healthcare Experience: Recommended

PA Shadowing: Recommended, not required

Required Standardized Testing: GRE

Letters of Recommendation: Three required; no one specific

Seat Deposit: None

CASPA Participant: Yes

Supplemental Application: No

Admissions: Not rolling

Application Deadline: September 1

Unique Program Features

Texas Preference: At least 90% of each class must come from Texas residents

Clinical Experiences: Students will experience clinical training at two new state-of-the-art on campus teaching hospitals and have opportunities for international clinical experiences.

Curriculum Focus: There is a focus and added emphasis on quality improvement and patient safety, with the developing opportunity for graduation with distinction in quality improvement and patient safety, providing an added value to employers.

UTAH

ROCKY MOUNTAIN UNIVERSITY OF HEALTH PROFESSIONS

Rocky Mountain University of Health Professions

122 East 1700 South
Provo, UT 84606
Phone: 801-375-5125
Email: pa@rmuohp.edu

PANCE Scores

5-year First Time Pass: N/A

Most Recent First Time Pass: N/A (have not graduated a class yet)

Mission: The mission of the RMUoHP PA Program is to educate competent physician assistant graduates who value and provide comprehensive, evidence-based, patient-centered care and who are committed to lifelong-learning, professional growth, and collaborative practice.

Curriculum Structure

Didactic: 14 months

Clinical: 14 months

Rotations: 8 mandatory, 1 elective, 1 inpatient selective, 4 weeks each

Accreditation: Provisional

Degree Offered: Master (MPAS)

Start Date: May annually

Program Length: 28 months

Class Capacity: 50 students

Tuition: $94,050

GPA Requirement: Overall GPA 3.2; Science GPA 3.2

Healthcare Experience: 250 hours required

PA Shadowing: Recommended

Required Standardized Testing: GRE (combined score of 298 and Analytical 3.5 is required)

Letters of Recommendation: Two required; no one specific

Seat Deposit: $500

Unique Program Features

Rotations: Students complete a primary care/family medicine rotation during their didactic year to break up the monotony of classes and begin to apply what they learn prior to full-time clinical rotations.

CASPA Participant: Yes

Supplemental Application: No

Admissions: Not specified

Application Deadline: October 1

Prerequisite Coursework

Human Anatomy with lab (3-4 credits), Human Physiology with lab (4 credits), General Biology with lab (4 credits), Microbiology with lab (4 credits), General Chemistry with lab (8-10 credits), Statistics (2-3 credits), College Algebra or higher (3 credits), Psychology (3 credits), Medical Terminology (1-3 credits). Anatomy, Physiology, Microbiology and Statistics must be completed in the last 10 years.

Class of 2017

Male: 43%
Female: 57%
Minority: 25%
GPA: 3.53
Science GPA: 3.48
GRE: not required
Faculty to Student Ratio: not reported
Average Healthcare Experience: 10,219 hours

PANCE Scores

5-year First Time Pass: 94%

Most Recent First Time Pass: 98%

Curriculum Structure

Didactic: 15 months
Clinical: 12 months
Rotations: 5 mandatory, 1 elective, variable duration

UNIVERSITY OF UTAH

University of Utah
Email: admissions@upap.utah.edu

375 Chipeta Way
Suite A
Salt Lake City, UT 84108
Phone: 801-581-7766

Mission: To increase access to health care, with a focus on medically underserved communities, by educating highly qualified physician assistants in the primary care model.

Accreditation: Continuing

Degree Offered: Master (MPAS)

Start Date: May annually

Program Length: 27 months

Class Capacity: 44 students

Tuition: In-state: $64,874; Out-of-state: $96,435

GPA Requirement: Overall GPA 2.7; Science GPA 2.7

Healthcare Experience: 2,000 hours required

PA Shadowing: Not required

Required Standardized Testing: None

Letters of Recommendation: Three required; no one specific

Seat Deposit: $1,000

CASPA Participant: Yes

Supplemental Application: Yes

Admissions: Not specified

Application Deadline: August 1

Unique Program Features

Admissions: Approximately 80% of each class is made up of Utah residents, while the other 20% comes from other states.

International Rotations: Students can choose to do a rotation in Thailand or Guatemala as an elective.

Community Engagement: Community Engagement at UPAP is a structured learning experience that combines community service with preparation and reflection. The focus is on critical, reflective thinking, civic responsibility, and commitment to the community. Students can complete opportunities at Head Start Migrant Farm Worker Program, Student-Run Free Clinic at Maliheh, and the Salt Lake Community Action Program.

Prerequisite Coursework

Human Anatomy with lab (4 credits), Human Physiology with lab (4 credits), Biology (4 credits), Chemistry (8 credits). Courses should be completed prior to September 15th of the application year.

VIRGINIA

EASTERN VIRGINIA MEDICAL SCHOOL

Eastern Virginia
Medical School
Email:
paprogram@evms.edu

651 Colley Avenue
3rd Floor
Norfolk, VA 23501
Phone: 757-446-7158

Mission: The mission of the EVMS Physician Assistant Program is to prepare students to provide health care in a broad range of medical settings by training them in the medical arts and sciences in an inclusive, multi-cultural environment dedicated to the delivery of patient centered care, while fostering a strong commitment to clinical and community partnerships.

Accreditation:
Continuing

Degree Offered:
Master (MPA)

Start Date:
January annually

Program Length:
28 months

Class Capacity:
80 students

Tuition:
In-state: $72,257;
Out-of-state: $82,484

GPA Requirement:
Overall GPA 3.0;
Prerequisite GPA 2.67

Healthcare Experience:
Preferred, not required

PA Shadowing: Not required

Required Standardized Testing: None

Letters of Recommendation: Three required; no one specific

Seat Deposit: $500

CASPA Participant: Yes

Supplemental Application: Yes

Admissions: Non-rolling

Application Deadline:
March 1

Class of 2018
Male: 21.7%
Female: 78.3%
Minority: 22.9%
GPA: 3.32
Prerequisite GPA: 3.82
GRE Total: 307
Faculty to Student Ratio: not reported
Average Healthcare Experience: 5,108 hours

PANCE Scores

5-year First Time Pass: 97%

Most Recent First Time Pass: 96%

Curriculum Structure
Didactic: 16 months
Clinical: 12 months
Rotations: 7 mandatory, 1 elective, 6 weeks each

Prerequisite Coursework

Anatomy, Physiology, General Chemistry, Organic Chemistry or Biochemistry, Microbiology or Cell Biology, Intro to Psychology, Additional Psychology, Math or Statistics or Physics. All must be completed with a B- or better by March 1. Science courses should be taken within the past 10 years.

Unique Program Features

Community Service: The program is very active in the community and has recently completed a project with elementary school students in conjunction with the United Way and Norfolk Public Schools.

Clinical Skills Curriculum: EVMS houses the Sentara Center for Simulation and Immersive Learning, which uses standardized patients in a controlled environment to teach clinical history taking and physical exam skills.

Class of 2017

Male: 7%

Female: 93%

Minority: 22.9%

GPA: 3.58

Science GPA: 3.53

GRE: not reported

Faculty to Student Ratio: not reported

Average Healthcare Experience: 4,037 hours

PANCE Scores

5-year First Time Pass: 93%

Most Recent First Time Pass: 100%

Curriculum Structure

Didactic: 16 months

Clinical: 12 months

Rotations: 9 mandatory, 1 elective, 1 research, 4 weeks each

Capstone Project: required for graduation

JAMES MADISON UNIVERSITY

James Madison University
Email: paprogram@jmu.edu

Physician Assistant Program
801 Carrier Drive, MSC 4301
Harrisonburg, VA 22807
Phone: 540-568-2395

Mission: The mission of the James Madison University Physician Assistant Program is to provide educational opportunities for students to develop the knowledge, skills, and attitudes necessary to function as primary care physician assistants, serving the medical needs of the Commonwealth of Virginia and society in general including rural and medically underserved areas.

Accreditation: Continuing

Degree Offered: Master (MPAS)

Start Date: August annually

Program Length: 28 months

Class Capacity: 30 students

Tuition:
In-state: $44,034;
Out-of-state: $86,428

GPA Requirement: No minimum

Healthcare Experience: 1,000 hours required

PA Shadowing: Not required

Required Standardized Testing: GRE

Letters of Recommendation: Three required; no one specific

Seat Deposit: $500

CASPA Participant: Yes

Supplemental Application: Yes

Admissions: Not specified

Application Deadline: September 1

Unique Program Features

Promotores de Salud: The PDS program trains Hispanic men and women to be health resource persons who are able to provide friends, family, and co-workers with culturally appropriate health information. JMU physician assistant students fill an integral role in the program by being the primary instructors of the 40-hour training. PA faculty act as resources providing academic support. PA students get the benefit of practicing presentation skills while also getting to experience working with Spanish interpreters.

Student Society: The student society at JMU is one of the most active in civic engagement and community service, recently having completed a variety of projects including a blood drive, road race, health fair, and blood pressure screenings.

Prerequisite Coursework

Human or Mammalian Physiology, Human or Mammalian Anatomy with lab, Biochemistry, Genetics, Microbiology, Medical Terminology. Aside from Medical Terminology, courses must have been completed in the last 7 years.

JEFFERSON COLLEGE OF HEALTH SCIENCES

Jefferson College of
Health Sciences
Email:
paadmissions@jchs.edu

—
101 Elm Avenue SE
Roanoke, VA 24013
Phone: 540-985-4016

PANCE Scores
5-year First Time Pass: 98%

Most Recent First Time Pass: 98%

Mission: The mission of the Jefferson College of Health Sciences Physician Assistant Program is to graduate competent and compassionate physician assistants who are well versed in the art and science of medicine and are prepared to effectively function as members of the healthcare team.

Curriculum Structure
Didactic: 14 months

Clinical: 13 months

Rotations: 10 mandatory, 2 elective, 4 weeks each

Master's Capstone: required for graduation

Accreditation: Continuing

Degree Offered: Master (MSPA)

Start Date: August annually

Program Length: 27 months

Class Capacity: 42 students

Tuition: $75,750

GPA Requirement: Overall GPA: 3.0

Healthcare Experience: 500 hours required

PA Shadowing: Not required

Required Standardized Testing: GRE

Letters of Recommendation: Three required; no one specific

Seat Deposit: $500

CASPA Participant: Yes

Supplemental Application: No

Admissions: Not specified

Application Deadline: November 1

Unique Program Features

Student Society: The student society at Jefferson is active in service learning activities, fundraises, professional advocacy activity, and attending the AAPA national conference each year.

Prerequisite Coursework

Anatomy and Physiology I and II with lab (8 credits), General Chemistry I and II with lab (8 credits), Biochemistry or Cell Biology (3 credits), Microbiology (4 credits), Genetics or Immunology (3 credits), Statistics (3 credits), Medical Terminology (1 credit), Psychology (6 credits, 1 course must be upper level). At least 12 hours of the coursework must have been completed in the past three years.

No class statistics reported

PANCE Scores

5-year First Time Pass: N/A

Most Recent First Time Pass: N/A (have not graduated a class)

Curriculum Structure

Didactic: 12 months

Clinical: 15 months (including summative)

Rotations: 7 mandatory, 2 elective, 2-8 weeks each

Master's Research: required for graduation

Unique Program Features

Facilities: The program boasts an anatomy lab featuring flat screen monitors and 21 cadaver stations as well as custom-designed PA program space in the Graduate Health Science Building which features advanced equipment and technology.

Doctoral Option: The program is developing a doctoral option where students who complete the MPAM program can engage in an additional 9 months of instruction to include a short clinical fellowship and coursework in leadership, healthcare management, organizational behavior, disaster medicine, and global health.

Lynchburg College
Email:
pa@lynchburg.edu

1501 Lakeside Drive
Lynchburg, VA 24501
Phone: 434-544-8876

Mission: The mission of the Lynchburg College Department of Physician Assistant Medicine is to educate Physician Assistants to become compassionate health care providers with an emphasis on teamwork, communication, human diversity and patient-centered care. The dynamic interdisciplinary advanced curriculum will facilitate the highest standard of patient care while also creating leaders within medicine, local and global communities, and accelerating the advancement of the profession.

Accreditation: Provisional

Degree Offered: Master (MPAM)

Start Date: June annually

Program Length: 27 months

Class Capacity: 30 students

Tuition: $79,772

GPA Requirement: Overall GPA: 3.0; Science GPA: 3.0; Prerequisite GPA 3.0

Healthcare Experience: 500 hours required

PA Shadowing: 8 hours required

Required Standardized Testing: GRE

Letters of Recommendation: Three required; One from a physician, PA, or NP

Seat Deposit: $1,000

CASPA Participant: Yes

Supplemental Application: Yes

Admissions: Rolling

Application Deadline: March 1

Prerequisite Coursework

Biology with lab (8 credits), General Chemistry or Introductory Chemistry with lab (4 credits), Organic Chemistry or Biochemistry with lab (4 credits), Human Anatomy and Physiology I and II with lab (8 credits), Microbiology with lab (3-4 credits), Genetics (3 credits), Psychology (3 credits), Statistics (3 credits), Social Sciences (3 credits).

MARY BALDWIN COLLEGE

Mary Baldwin College/
Murphy Deming
College of Health
Sciences

100 Baldwin Boulevard
Fishersville, VA 22939
Phone: 540-887-4000
Email: MDCHSadmit@mbc.edu

Mission: The mission of the Physician Assistant (PA) Program at Mary Baldwin College is to academically and clinically prepare students for the practice of medicine as compassionate, effective, well-qualified physician assistants able to serve in a variety of medical specialty areas and settings under the direction and supervision of a licensed physician.

Accreditation:
Provisional

Degree Offered:
Master (MSPA)

Start Date:
January annually

Program Length:
27 months

Class Capacity:
45 students

Tuition: $80,570

GPA Requirement:
Overall GPA: 3.0

Healthcare Experience:
Recommended, not required

PA Shadowing: Not required

Required Standardized Testing: GRE or MCAT

Letters of Recommendation: Three required; no one specific

Seat Deposit: $1,500

CASPA Participant: Yes

Supplemental Application: No

Admissions: Not specified

Application Deadline: October 1

Prerequisite Coursework

Biology with lab (3-4 credits), Human or Vertebrate Anatomy with lab (3-4 credits), Human or Vertebrate Physiology with lab (3-4 credits), Microbiology with lab (3-4 credits), Chemistry with lab (3-4 credits), Organic Chemistry or Biochemistry (3-4 credits), Psychology (6 credits, 1 must be an upper level course), Statistics (3 credits), Medical Terminology (1-2 credits). All courses must be completed prior to September 1 other than Medical Terminology.

No class statistics reported

PANCE Scores

5-year First Time Pass: N/A

Most Recent First Time Pass: N/A (have not graduated a class)

Curriculum Structure

Didactic: 15 months

Clinical: 12 months

Rotations:
7 mandatory,
2 elective,
4-8 weeks each

Unique Program Features

Facilities: The new Health Sciences Building is a three-story facility that is the flagship building in Fishersville, Virginia. Completed in June 2014, this facility includes four large classrooms; six seminar rooms; nine clinical laboratories, including a simulation suite; two research spaces; faculty/staff offices and numerous collaborative learning spaces.

Students: Though Mary Baldwin was traditionally an all-girls school, it has accepted both male and female students into its graduate programs for approximately 30 years. They are also a military friendly institution.

PANCE Scores

5-year First Time Pass: 99%

Most Recent First Time Pass: 100%

Curriculum Structure

Didactic: 18 months

Clinical: 12 months

Rotations:
7 mandatory,
1 elective,
1 community preceptorship
4-8 weeks each

Prerequisite Coursework

Human Anatomy and Physiology with lab (8 credits), General or Introductory Chemistry with lab (4 credits), Biochemistry (4 credits), Microbiology with lab (4 credits), Abnormal Psychology (3 credits), Child Developmental or Life Span Psychology (3 credits), Mathematics (3 credits), Medical Terminology (3 credits). Courses should be taken within the last 10 years.

SHENANDOAH UNIVERSITY

Shenandoah University
Email: pa@su.edu

1460 University Drive
Winchester, VA 22601
Phone: 540-542-6208

Mission: The mission of the Shenandoah University Division of Physician Assistant Studies is to provide a comprehensive educational program in a collaborative and supportive environment to develop highly skilled, well-educated, compassionate primary-care oriented physician assistants who are capable of providing high quality, patient-centered health care in a variety of settings.

Accreditation: Continuing

Degree Offered: Master (MPAS)

Start Date: July annually

Program Length: 30 months

Class Capacity: 42 students

Tuition: $71,380

GPA Requirement:
Overall GPA: 3.0;
Science GPA: 3.0

Healthcare Experience: Recommended, not required

PA Shadowing: Not required

Required Standardized Testing: GRE

Letters of Recommendation: Three required; no one specific

Seat Deposit: $500

CASPA Participant: Yes

Supplemental Application: No

Admissions: Rolling

Application Deadline: January 15

Unique Program Features

Medical Mission Trip: Over 50% of each class participates in a medical mission trip to Nicaragua where students provide medical care in three different rural clinics.

Performing Arts Medicine: PA students have the opportunity to earn a certificate in Performing Arts Medicine through the Division of athletic training.

Expansion: The program is planning to expand to a second location in Leesburg, VA. The SU PA program will operate under the philosophy of two campuses, one class, one faculty. The curriculum will be delivered synchronously utilizing distance learning technology between both campuses and the program will work to ensure equity between the two campuses.

WASHINGTON

HERITAGE UNIVERSITY

Heritage University

Email:
PA_HU@heritage.edu

3240 Fort Road
Toppenish, WA 98948
Phone: Not provided

Mission: The mission of the Physician Assistant Educational Program at Heritage is to increase access to healthcare, particularly in the rural or underserved areas of the Pacific Northwest, by educating future Physician Assistants who will provide high quality medical care in a compassionate and competent manner.

Accreditation:
Provisional

Degree Offered:
Master (MSPA)

Start Date:
May annually

Program Length:
24 months

Class Capacity:
32 students

Tuition: $78,400

GPA Requirement:
Overall GPA 2.75;
Science GPA 3.0;
Prerequisite GPA 3.0

Healthcare Experience:
1,000 hours required

PA Shadowing: Not required

Required Standardized Testing: None

Letters of Recommendation: Three required; one from a PA, one from a physician, one from a supervisor.

Seat Deposit: $500

CASPA Participant: Yes

Supplemental Application: Yes

Admissions: Rolling

Application Deadline:
November 1

Prerequisite Coursework

Anatomy and Physiology I and II (6 credits), Microbiology with lab (3 credits), Human Sciences (6 credits), Math (3 credits). All should be completed by January 1 of the year you are applying to enter.

Unique Program Features

Rural and Underserved Focus: Most rotations take place in rural or underserved communities, primarily in Washington, Oregon, Idaho, Montana and Alaska. Most of these learning centers are based in small towns that have smaller hospitals with active emergency departments, a few key specialists, and a good family medicine or internal medicine base.

Continuity Clinic: The clinical phase is integrated so that students spend 2-3 days each week in a family medicine environment and the other days in specialty settings.

Class of 2016
Male: 51%
Female: 49%
GPA: 3.35
Military Background: 27.5%

PANCE Scores
5-year First Time Pass: 86%

Most Recent First Time Pass: varies by campus

Curriculum Structure
Didactic: 13 months
Clinical: 13 months
Rotations: 6 mandatory, 1 elective, 1 month each except family medicine (4 months)
Capstone Project: required for graduation

Unique Program Features
One Program, Four Campuses: The MCHS students are accepted in either Seattle, WA or Spokane, WA while the BCHS students are located in Tacoma, WA and Anchorage, AK. Each has its own unique lifestyle and vibe.

Rural and Underserved Focus: The program trains students in primary care in rural and underserved areas. Students complete a four month family medicine rotation and travel to different sites to work with a variety of populations.

UNIVERSITY OF WASHINGTON

University of Washington
Email:
medex@uw.edu

4311 11th Avenue NE
Ste. 200
Seattle, WA 98105
Phone: 206-616-4001

Mission: MEDEX Northwest is a regional program that educates physician assistants in a proven tradition of excellence. MEDEX Northwest, the University of Washington School of Medicine's Physician Assistant Program, is committed to educating experienced health personnel from diverse backgrounds to practice medicine with physician supervision. The program provides a broad, competency-based curriculum that focuses on primary care with an emphasis on underserved populations. MEDEX encourages life-long learning to meet ever-changing health care needs. As a pioneer in PA education, MEDEX continues to be innovative in identifying, creating, and filling new niches for PAs as a strategy for expanding health care access.

Accreditation: Continued

Degree Offered: Bachelor (BCHS), Master (MCHS)

Start Date: July annually

Program Length: 26 months

Class Capacity: 140 students

Tuition: Bachelor: 59,509; Master:$71,710

GPA Requirement: Prerequisite GPA: 2.7

Healthcare Experience: 2,000 hours required

PA Shadowing: Not required

Required Standardized Testing: GRE (MCHS only)

Letters of Recommendation: Three required; one from a PA, one from a physician, one from a supervisor.

Seat Deposit: $500

CASPA Participant: Yes
Supplemental Application: Yes

Admissions: Rolling
Application Deadline: October 1

Prerequisite Coursework
Human Anatomy and Physiology I and II (6 credits), General Biology (3 credits), Microbiology (3 credits), Chemistry (3 credits), Statistics (3 credits), English (6 credits). All must be completed by the application deadline with a B- or better.

WISCONSIN

CARROLL UNIVERSITY

Carroll University
Email:
painfo@carrollu.edu

100 N. East Avenue
Waukesha, WI 53186
Phone: 262-524-7361

Mission: The Mission of the Master of Science in Physician Assistant Studies Program is to educate physician assistants to provide comprehensive quality health care to all, respectful of patient/client values, committed to ethical principles and grounded in evidence-based practice and clinical reasoning. Graduates will contribute to the profession and communities and be prepared to practice medicine in a variety of primary care settings under the supervision of physicians. Graduates will also be prepared to provide service to medically underserved communities and diverse patient populations.

Accreditation:
Continued

Degree Offered:
Master (MSPAS)

Start Date:
June annually

Program Length:
24 months

Class Capacity:
20 students

Tuition: $63,360

CASPA Participant:
Yes

Supplemental Application: Yes

Admissions:
Not specified

Application Deadline: October 1

GPA Requirement:
Overall GPA 3.0;
Science GPA 3.0;

Healthcare Experience:
250 hours required

PA Shadowing: not required

Required Standardized Testing: GRE

Letters of Recommendation: Three required; preferably from a college instructor, a supervisor from a work or volunteer clinical experience, and a health care professional such as PA, NP, MD or DO

Seat Deposit: $500

Class of 2017
Male: 25%
Female: 75%
Minority: not reported
GPA: 3.76
Science GPA: 3.70
GRE Quantitative: 63rd percentile
GRE Verbal: 59th percentile
GRE Analytical: not reported
Faculty to Student Ratio: not reported
Average Healthcare Experience: 2,130 hours

PANCE Scores
5-year First Time Pass: 98% (based on 3 years of data)

Most Recent First Time Pass: 95%

Curriculum Structure
Didactic: 12 months
Clinical: 12 months
Rotations: 7 mandatory, 1 elective, 2-8 weeks each
Capstone Project: required for graduation

Prerequisite Coursework

Anatomy, Physiology, Microbiology, Other Biological Sciences (2 semesters), Chemistry (4 semesters), Psychology (2 semesters), Statistics. Anatomy and Physiology must be taken within five years of admission to the program and should be completed prior to application.

Unique Program Features

Early Clinical Exposure: Exposure in the first year provides students with hands-on patient/client experience that allows students to integrate classroom learning with practical and clinical applications while providing service to the community and help students develop clinical skills, and emphasize wellness and prevention across the lifespan.

Admissions Preference: Carroll graduates receive additional points towards admission during the admissions process. Approximately 12-20% of students are prior Carroll graduates per year.

PANCE Scores

5-year First Time Pass: 98% (based on 3 years of data)

Most Recent First Time Pass: N/A (have not graduated a class yet)

Curriculum Structure

Didactic: 14 months

Clinical: 12 months

Rotations: 9 mandatory, 2 elective, 4 weeks each

Unique Program Features

Admissions Preference: Current Concordia students or graduates who have a cumulative GPA of 3.4 and science prerequisite GPA of 3.40 will be guaranteed an interview.

Primary Care Focus: This program has a focus on primary care, preventive medicine, and health literacy and students will work with a variety of primary care and medically underserved populations.

CONCORDIA UNIVERSITY

Concordia University
Email: renee.knuth@cuw.edu

12800 N. Lake Shore Drive
Mequon, WI 53097
Phone: 262-243-4437

Mission: The Physician Assistant program at CUW prepares students to become competent physician assistants who provide quality health care in a respectful, culturally sensitive, caring and knowledgeable manner. CUW PA graduates are committed to caring for patients in mind, body and spirit with an emphasis on primary care and preventive medicine as well as continual lifelong learning.

Accreditation: Provisional

Degree Offered: Master (MSPAS)

Start Date: May annually

Program Length: 26 months

Class Capacity: 30 students

Tuition: $75,920

CASPA Participant: Yes

Supplemental Application: No

Admissions: Rolling

Application Deadline: September 1

GPA Requirement: Overall GPA 3.0; Science GPA 3.0; Prerequisite GPA 3.0

Healthcare Experience: 100 hours required

PA Shadowing: 24 hours required

Required Standardized Testing: None

Letters of Recommendation: Three required; two professional or academic, one from a PA, NP, DO, or MD that has worked with the applicant in a patient care setting.

Seat Deposit: $500

Prerequisite Coursework

General Chemistry I and II with lab, Biochemistry, Microbiology, Human Anatomy and Physiology I and II with lab, Genetics, Biology (2 semesters) with lab, Psychology, Statistics, College Algebra or higher, Medical Terminology. Anatomy and Physiology must be taken within five years of applying to the program.

MARQUETTE UNIVERSITY

Marquette University
Email:
doris.osterhaus.
marquette.edu

1700 W. Wells Street
Milwaukee, WI 53233
Phone: 414-288-5688

Mission: The Department of Physician Assistant Studies combines Marquette's Jesuit tradition of cura personalis ("care for the whole person") with the College of Health Sciences' Jesuit ideals of concern for the spiritual, emotional and physical development of the individual. We're dedicated to educating physician assistants for supervised practice in dynamic health care systems. We realize our mission through a synergistic strategy of educational goals.

Accreditation:
Continuing

Degree Offered:
Master (MSPAS)

Start Date:
August annually

Program Length:
33 months

Class Capacity:
55 students

Tuition: $94,377

GPA Requirement:
Overall GPA 3.0;

Healthcare Experience:
200 hours required

PA Shadowing: Not required

Required Standardized Testing: GRE

Letters of Recommendation: Three required; no one specific

Seat Deposit: $1,000

CASPA Participant: Yes

Supplemental Application: Yes

Admissions: Not specified

Application Deadline:
October 1

Prerequisite Coursework

Biology (2 semesters), General Chemistry with lab (4 credits), Biochemistry, Social Science, Statistics, Medical Terminology. Highly recommended that course be completed in the last 5 years and taken at a 4-year institution.

No class statistics reported

PANCE Scores
5-year First Time Pass: 100%

Most Recent First Time Pass: 100%

Curriculum Structure
Didactic: 21 months
Clinical: 12 months
Rotations:
7 mandatory,
3 elective,
3-6 weeks each

Unique Program Features

Admissions Preference: Approximately 50% of each class is chosen from Marquette undergraduate students, while 50% is chosen from external candidates.

Clinical Rotations: Nationwide relationships with preceptors for rotations both in the US and abroad. Recently, students have traveled to Belize for rotation work.

Biomedical Sciences Curriculum: The didactic curriculum is 20 months long allowing for in depth study of biomedical sciences at a manageable pace with more time for synthesis than other programs.

UNIVERSITY OF WISCONSIN — LA CROSSE

University of Wisconsin
Email:
paprogram@uwlax.edu

1725 State Street
Health Science Center 4033
La Crosse, WI 54601
Phone: 608-785-6624

Mission: The mission of our program is to educate highly competent and compassionate physician assistants who excel in meeting the healthcare needs of the regions served by the partner institutions.

Accreditation: Continuing

Degree Offered: Master (MSPAS)

Start Date: May annually

Program Length: 24 months

Class Capacity: 19 students

Tuition: In-state $42,813; Out-of-state: $79,671

GPA Requirement: Overall GPA 3.0; Science GPA 3.0

Healthcare Experience: Expected, not required

PA Shadowing: Not required

Required Standardized Testing: GRE

Letters of Recommendation: Three required; no one specific

Seat Deposit: $500

CASPA Participant: Yes

Supplemental Application: Yes

Admissions: Not specified

Application Deadline: August 1

Prerequisite Coursework

Human Anatomy and Physiology I and II, Microbiology, Health Related Upper Division Biological Science (at least 14 total biology credits with 2 lab courses), General Chemistry, Organic Chemistry, Biochemistry (at least 11 total chemistry credits with 2 lab courses), Precalculus or Calculus, Statistics, Psychology.

Unique Program Features

Clinical Affiliation: The program is affiliated with the May Clinic Health System and students complete several rotations at the Mayo Clinic and associated facilities.

Facilities: The Health Science Center serves at the PA Program home with space for didactic lectures, exam rooms, and a study lounge. It is home to the Medical Dosimetry Program, Occupational Therapy Program, Physical Therapy Program, and Radiation Therapy Program.

Admissions Preference: Keeping in line with the program mission, the program aims to accept applicants who plan to work in the Wisconsin and Minnesota areas.

UNIVERSITY OF WISCONSIN – MADISON

University of Wisconsin
Email: paprogram@mailplus.wisc.edu

750 Highland Avenue
Health Science Learning Center RM 1278
Madison, WI 53705
Phone: 608-263-5620

PANCE Scores
5-year First Time Pass: 97%

Most Recent First Time Pass: 97%

Curriculum Structure
Didactic: 12 months

Clinical: 12 months

Rotations: 4 mandatory, 4 elective, 4-8 weeks each

Capstone Project: required for graduation

Mission: The mission of the University of Wisconsin-Madison Physician Assistant Program is to educate professionals committed to the delivery of comprehensive health care in a culturally and ethnically sensitive manner, with an emphasis on primary health care for populations and regions in need.

Accreditation: Continuing

Degree Offered: Master (MPAS)

Start Date: May annually

Program Length: 24 months

Class Capacity: 50 students

Tuition: In-state $35,031; Out-of-state: $71,680

GPA Requirement: Overall GPA 3.0; Science GPA 3.0

Healthcare Experience: 500 hours required

PA Shadowing: Not required

Required Standardized Testing: None

Letters of Recommendation: Three required; no one specific

Seat Deposit: None

CASPA Participant: Yes

Supplemental Application: Yes

Admissions: Not specified

Application Deadline: September 1

Prerequisite Coursework
Mammalian Biology with lab, Microbiology with lab, Biochemistry, Human Anatomy, Human Physiology, Statistics, Psychology. Anatomy and Physiology must be taken within 3 years of matriculation.

Unique Program Features

Distance Education Option: The program offers a 3 year distance education option with 2 years of part time didactic work and 1 year of full time clinical work in the students home community. It is generally reserved for students who have a desire to practice in their home rural or underserved community.

Dual Degree: Students can complete a dual degree MPH/PA program where the first year consists of MPH coursework and the 2nd and 3rd years comprise the PA program.

wisPACT: There is a northern Wisconsin community track option where students attend live lectures and discussions via video conferencing at UW-Marathon County as well. It is generally reserved for those who want to practice in northern Wisconsin.

Student Testimonials: These are available on the website for applicants to get an insider perspective on the program.

Made in the USA
Lexington, KY
15 July 2016